TEARS & TRIUMPHS

A look into the world of children with
Down Syndrome or other Developmental Delays

VALENTINE DMITRIEV PH.D.

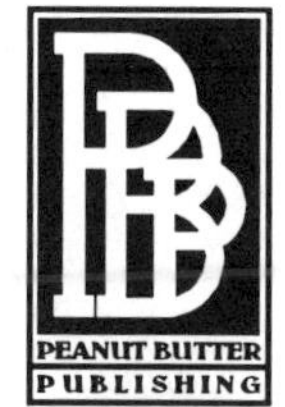

Seattle, Washington
Portland, Oregon
Denver, Colorado
Vancouver, B.C.

Cover Photo:
Patrick Evezich receives his diploma from C. Richard Ellis, principal of Eastside Catholic High School

ISBN 0-89716-715-5
LOC
A1.0057
Cover design: David Marty
Editing & Production: Elizabeth Lake

First printing May 1997
10 9 8 7 6 5 4 3 2 1

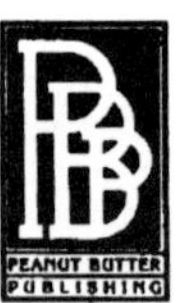

Peanut Butter Publishing
226 2nd Avenue West • Seattle, WA 98119
(206) 281-5965 • FAX (206) 281-5969
Portland, OR (503) 222-5527 • Denver, CO (303) 322-0065
Vancouver, B.C. (604) 688-0320 • Scottsdale, AZ (602) 947-3575
e mail: pnutpub@aol.com
WWW home page: http://www.pbpublishing.com

Printed in the United States of America

Dedication

To Nick: in loving memory.
1906-1990

Table of Contents

Acknowledgements

I wish to thank Sidney W. Bijou, Judy Marick, Patricia Oelwein, Elizabeth Lake, Kathleen M. Isaac and David Marty for their professional assistance. I also wish to thank all the parents and children who enriched my life, challenged and inspired me.

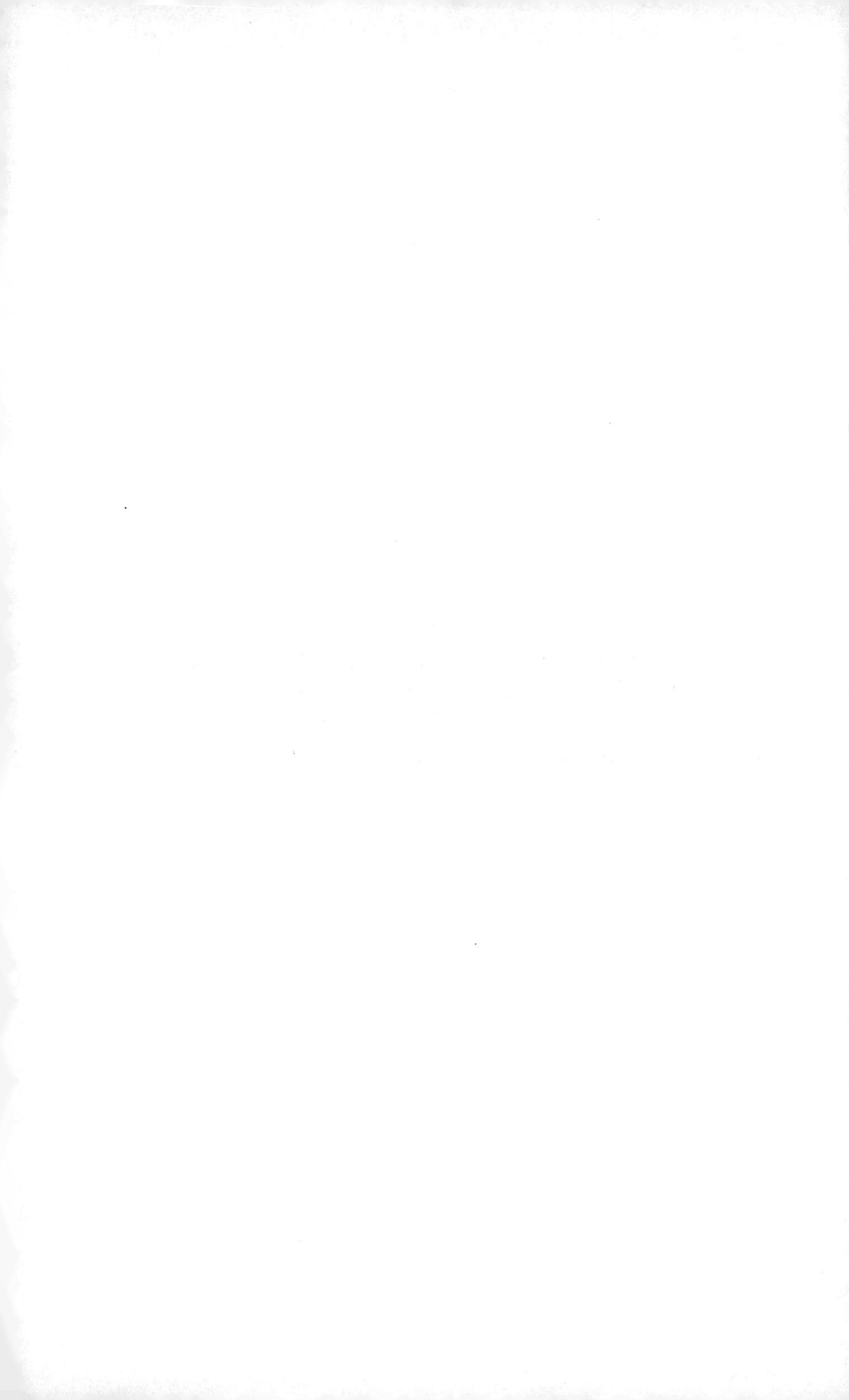

Foreword

This volume gives an excellent account of what can be done by a person dedicated to helping children develop, particularly those with Down syndrome. Dr. Dmitriev's case studies clearly show that behaviorally oriented early intervention in the hands of a dedicated person can encourage children with Down syndrome to develop beyond traditional expectations and bring joy and happiness to them and their parents. In a way, *Tears and Triumphs* not only describes the emotional vicissitudes of the children and their parents in the program, but also Dr. Dmitriev's own dark and sunny days. Her struggles were grounded not only in the problems of creating new treatment programs, but also in dealing with persons with preconceived ideas about the limitations of children with Down Syndrome.

In the course of sharing her many exciting experiences with the reader, she pauses now and then to emphasize some of the important lessons learned. For example, she reminds workers in adoption agencies about the need to be particularly careful in selecting potential parents for children with developmental disabilities; she advises parents to be persistent and assertive in seeking adequate diagnoses for any physical condition of their children; and she tells teachers that effective early intervention requires an empirically based curriculum and teaching method. No wonder her work quickly attracted the attention of parents, special educators, and other professionals around the world.

Another interesting feature of this volume is Dr. Dmetriev's account of how she came to devote herself to the education and treatment of children with Down Syndrome. The turning point in her career occurred when she decided that she must return to school for additional training if she were going to be effective in helping children with Down syndrome. It so happened that the first course she took at the University of Washington was a summer course given by Dr. Barbara Etzel at the Rainier State School at Buckley, Washington. Dr. Etzel, who was a professor of psychology at Western Washington University at that time, gave a course in the behavior analysis of child development in conjunction with the faculty of the University of Washington's Institute of Child Development of which I was the director. At that time the staffs of the three divisions of the Institute — nursery school, child clinic, and research laboratory — were introducing innovative research, teaching, and demonstration programs. What was new and different was that all of the work was based on the principles of behavior which had evolved from over 40 years of psychological research and a naturalistic philosophy of science.

One of the demonstrations was the Experimental Class at the Rainier State School to which Dr. Dmitriev alluded. This project came about after I personally surveyed a number of publicized programs for young handicapped children in the Boston area, and came to the conclusion that a program based on behavioral principles would be more effective than anything I had seen or read about. With the approval and support of the superintendent of the Rainier State School, Dr. Wesley White, a special classroom was constructed so that instruction in reading, writing, and arithmetic was to be completely individualized. It was the responsibility of two behaviorally trained teachers to conduct the class, and at the same time, to devise a hierarchical sequence of basic tasks to be taught (curriculum), to develop a record-keeping system that would assure that each child was always working at his or her level of competence, to devise an effective motivational system, and to establish teaching procedures based on behavior principles. The results were gratifying: the children not only made good progress but they enjoyed their experience in the classroom.

Another demonstration project referred to by Dr. Dmitriev was a special preschool class for children with behavior and emotional problems. Here the aim was to use behavioral principles and recording procedures to reduce problem behavior, such as excessive aggression, and at the same time to enhance development. It was in this program that Dr. Dmitriev received one-to-one training under the supervision of Florence Harris, Director of the Nursery School, and other members of the Institute staff.

The work at the Institute and the laboratory at the Rainier State School resulted in a flow of publications and presentations at professional meetings. Before long educators and clinical psychologists in this country were applying the same principles and method in special education classes (e.g., the engineered classroom in Los Angeles); for training parents to work with own handicapped children in their homes (e.g., the Portage Project for home teaching); to the treatment of children with autism (e.g., the autism program in the

Psychology Department of the University of California at Los Angeles); to the auxiliary treatment of children with life-threatening medical conditions (e.g., the program for hospitalized, terminally-ill children with cancer); and to Dr. Dmitriev's program for children with Down syndrome. The approach also "caught on" in countries abroad: in Japan (e.g., the Portage Project for home teaching); in Peru (e.g., Ann Sullivan Center for Special Education); in England (e.g., The Portage Project for home teaching); in Italy (e.g., the first book for teachers and parents on the education of children with retarded development); in Spain (e.g., a university clinic for children with behavior problems); in Venezuela (e.g., establishment of a child study laboratory at the Central University of Venezuela); and in Mexico (e.g., a private school for normally developing children in Hermosillo).

It would be misleading to say that these programs were productive and effective solely because the teachers and psychologists were trained in the application of behavior principles either directly or through the literature. Two other ingredients were necessary: they had to believe, as Dr. Dmitriev did, that each and every child they worked with had a real potential for growth and development and they had to be sensitive and flexible in their application of the principles.

Dr. Dmitriev's account of the treatment of children with Down syndrome, and the the education and treatment programs mentioned above, represent only the beginning of what can be accomplished. Since the behavioral approach is constantly being expanded and refined through research, teachers and clinicians in the future will be trained to be even better equipped to help all children with developmental disabilities and their parents as well.

Sidney W. Bijou, Ph. D.

Preface

Based upon case histories, *Tears and Triumphs* is about the sorrows, triumphs, courage and dedication of parents whose children happened to be born with physical and mental disabilities. It is also a record of the dramatic changes that have occurred in education, medicine and the general public's awareness and acceptance of the disabled.

As an educator with a Ph.D. in Early Childhood Special Education I have worked with these families, sharing their tears and moments of rejoicing for over thirty years; and I have witnessed and even played a part in fostering these attitudinal changes.

Although some of the children under my care were impaired as a result of brain damage or other nongenetic causes, the majority had been born with Down syndrome. This, unfortunately, is an exceedingly common abnormality. Among normal babies, one out of every 1000 is born with Down syndrome.

In the past, some twenty-five years ago, it was falsely believed that a child born with Down syndrome would be profoundly retarded, unable to attain anything resembling normal development. The majority of these infants were institutionalized, and parents viewed the birth of such a baby as the greatest calamity of their lives. Regretfully even today some people are influenced by these erroneous beliefs.

Although Down syndrome cannot be cured, a great deal can be done medically and educationally to overcome many of the physical and mental problems associated with this anomaly. Present day research has established, in fact, that children with Down syndrome can learn and can develop. In many instances their progress exceeds our highest expectations. The key to this achievement lies in early intervention. Early-enriching experiences are essential for the environment must now compensate for congenital or acquired disabilities. Through systematic, data-based, goal-oriented instruction, developmentally delayed children can learn skills which will enable them to function adequately in the environment, to achieve a higher quality of life as well as social acceptance in spite of their differences. This approach to education has successfully reversed the previous pessimistic view of these children's future, especially in the case of Down syndrome. The medical profession has also made great progress in the diagnosis, treatment and prevention of health problems associated with this anomaly.

It must be recognized that none of these advances would have been possible without the efforts of researchers and educators who had the vision and courage to introduce innovative educational programs based upon principles of behavior and scientific methodology. Such pioneer work demonstrated that instruction based upon these principles could not only modify undesirable behaviors among developmentally delayed children, but could also successfully teach them academic, functional and vocational skills.

Much of this early experimental work was conducted at the University of Washington in Seattle, and I wish to pay tribute to those who were destined to teach me and change my life and indirectly the lives of children and parents with whom I became involved. I specifically wish to thank Dr. Sidney W. Bijou, my mentor, as well as his colleagues Donald M. Baer, Montrose M. Wolf, Charles H. Strother, Norris G Haring and Alice H. Hayden.

Finally, *Tears and Triumphs* traces my own personal journey as a wife, mother, student and educator. The stories are true, only the names, except in specific instances, have been changed. Asterisks identify actual names when they appear for the first time.

Valentine Dmitriev, Ph.D.

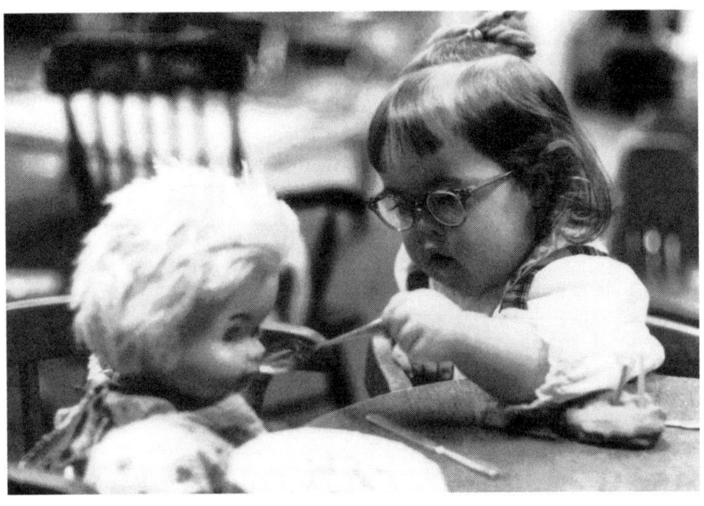

Maggie "feeds" her dolls in the housekeeping play area.

Chapter One
Phone Calls

I was sitting in my office, charting the progress of a developmentally disabled infant, when the phone rang. Picking up the receiver, I gave my name.

Silence.

Then I heard the rasping sounds of bitter weeping.

"How can I help you?" I asked.

"My daughter," a woman spoke, disjointed words spurting through her sobs. "My beautiful daughter gave birth to ... a ... " she whispered a fearful word, squeezing it through clenched teeth, *"Mongoloid!"*

An infant with Down syndrome; I understood. My heart reached out to the distraught grandmother.

"When was the baby born?"

"This morning, at seven-thirty."

I glanced at the clock behind my desk. That was less than three hours ago, so the pain was fresh, the wound raw and bleeding.

"I ... I knew a mongoloid boy once," the woman continued. "I was just a child then, but I remember so clearly. He lived in our neighborhood. It was terrible, terrible. He was a clumsy boy, ten or twelve years old. His nose was always running, he never used a handkerchief, his tongue hung out, he couldn't speak, he could hardly walk and he messed in his pants! Oh, what can we do!" Renewed sobs vibrated over the wire.

"A great deal can be done for children with Down syndrome," I replied. "What you describe happened many years ago. It's different now. We don't even use the term mongoloid anymore."

Now was 1973, five years since I initiated an experimental program for children with Down syndrome. Funded by the Department of Health, Education and Welfare, we were housed at the Experimental Education Unit of the Child Development and Mental Retardation Center at the University of Washington in Seattle, Washington.[1] Thinking about the fifty Down syndrome youngsters currently enrolled in our infant, toddler, preschool and kindergarten classes, and the progress these so-called hopelessly retarded children were making, it was easy to give positive reassurance. I ended our conversation with an invitation to visit our model classrooms.

Mrs. Miles arrived a few days later. I met her in the front lobby and escorted her to an observation booth, a small room adjoining the classroom. A one-way mirror enabled us to observe, unseen, without distracting the children. We saw twelve three-year-olds happily engaged in various preschool activities. Two boys, draped in long aprons were easel painting, smiling and nudging each other as they dipped their brushes into jars of red, blue or yellow paint. Another group of preschoolers stood at a water table, floating boats and plastic toys and pouring cupfuls of water to activate the mechanism of water wheel. Seated apart, in a secluded corner, a teacher and an attentive child with pink ribbons in her hair worked on a color recognition task.

A student teacher and the remaining children were gathered around a table. They were working with puzzles and nesting blocks. Three women, mothers, who had been scheduled to participate in the classroom this day, moved about unobtrusively, stepping in to assist a child when necessary.

Several minutes passed as Mrs. Miles watched in silence. Finally she turned and whispered:

"Where are the mongoloid children?"

"You're looking at them," I replied.

"But they look so normal!"

"Yes, they do," I smiled, "yet, every one of these children has Down syndrome."

She shook her head in disbelief. "Then Charlie, my little grandson could ... ?"

"Of course. But you must begin his program as soon as possible. Come, let's visit the infant class."

Mothers, and sometimes fathers, brought their babies to the Infant Program once a week. During the one hour session a teacher, trained in early child development, worked with the child, demonstrating various exercises. Based upon patterns of normal growth, the exercises taught fundamental skills which normal babies acquire spontaneously. The youngest infants practiced neck and upper body control, as well as fixating and tracking by following moving objects with their eyes. Older children learned how to grasp toys, how to roll over and how to sit without support. At the end of the session parents were instructed in how to continue the exercises at home.

When we left the classroom, Mrs. Miles's eyes were glowing, her face looked flushed with excitement and she was smiling.

"That's how I played with my daughter when she was a baby!"

"Exactly," I agreed. "Many of the activities are based on what parents do instinctively."

"Then why," she questioned, "do we need infant learning programs?"

I responded by explaining that parents of impaired infants are often stymied, they are depressed, afraid to try, easily discouraged if their baby is unable to master a new skill right away. Parental play time is vital to the development of all babies, and its importance should not be overlooked. Nevertheless, in order to minimize inherent deficiencies, infants with disabilities require the additional benefits of a structured program, designed to meet specific needs.

"But we live so far away, more than a hundred miles from Seattle! Where will we find a program for Charlie? She bit her lip and turned aside, fighting a new rush of tears.

"We'll work it out," I promised, and we did.

Charlie and his parents came to the Unit for an initial assessment. His developmental program was outlined; his parents were given a set of written instructions and shown how to continue the procedures at home. From then on we monitored Charlie's progress once a month. The last time I saw Charlie he was two years old. He walked into the classroom, a sturdy, self-assured youngster. He gave me a bright smile, said, "Hi," then walked over to the book case and pulled down a picture book. Sitting down on the floor, he began turning the pages.

Mrs. Miles squeezed my hand. "Isn't he wonderful! I'm so proud of Charlie, and my daughter and son-in-law. They're marvelous parents and I can't believe that I'm the same hysterical woman who telephoned you two years ago!"

" I'm glad you did."

"Oh, so am I!"

A few weeks later I received a letter from Mrs. Miles. She thanked me again for the help I had given Charlie and his family and then added that her daughter was expecting another baby, a normal little girl, as confirmed by amniocentesis. Amniocentesis is a prenatal diagnostic procedure performed to determine whether or not the developing fetus will have Down syndrome or some other abnormality. Between the fourteenth and sixteenth weeks of pregnancy a sample of fetal cells is obtained from the amniotic fluid which surrounds the baby in the womb. A thin needle, passed through the abdomen, collects the liquid which contains loose cells shed by the skin of the fetus. The sample cells are then placed in culture tubes and allowed to grow for several weeks. After the cells have multiplied sufficiently the chromosomes in the cells are studied and identified. It is then possible to make a diagnosis.

It should be remembered that the cells in an individual with Down syndrome contain forty-seven chromosomes, whereas normal human cells have only forty-six. The amniocentesis performed on Charlie's mother and the subsequent analysis showed that the sample cells had the desired number of forty-six chromosomes, confirming that her unborn baby was normal. This test also determines the sex of a fetus, thus it was revealed that Mrs. Miles' grandchild would be a girl.

It is strongly recommended that every pregnant woman at risk of delivering a child with Down syndrome, or with some other genetic defect, as for example, spina bifida, an extremely serious orthopedic disorder, seek prebirth diagnosis either through amniocentesis or by a chorionic villi sampling. In this procedure tissue representative of the fetus is obtained from the uterus wall where the future placenta is forming.

The sample is obtained by passing a catheter through the cervix into the uterus.[2]

The letter from Mrs. Miles brought other exciting news. In a few days Charlie would begin attending a toddler group for normal children, and she, herself, was taking a course in child development at the local community college.

"I want to work with handicapped children," she wrote, "and of course I want to keep up with Charlie. Am I too old to begin a new career at forty-nine?"

The ease with which Charlie's family adjusted to his presence was fairly typical. Most parents, after the initial shock, quickly learn to love and accept their imperfect infants. Nevertheless, there are those who are emotionally unable to make this transition. Their rejection is so complete that it's futile to hope for acceptance. Maggie's father was such a man.

MAGGIE

The man had a harsh voice. "Is this the place for mongoloids?" he demanded over the phone.

"Yes," I responded, "We have a program for children with Down syndrome."

"I mean do you keep them?"

"I'm not sure that I understand your question," I apologized.

"One of those mongoloids was born to my wife three days ago. Well, I don't want it. What I need to know is, do you keep them?"

"This is a school, not an institution. We don't *keep* children here."

"There must be some place that does. What about a State school?"

"Institutions no longer accept infants."

"So what am I going to do? I told you I don't want it! "

"What about your wife? How does she feel about this?"

I heard a woman's low voice in the background, then the man's sharp response, "All right!"

He came back on the line. "She wants to talk to you in person."

"Of course. I'll be glad to meet with your wife, with both of you. I could see her at the hospital if she wishes, or you could make an appointment to come here."

"How about now, in half an hour. I'm checking her out of the hospital in a few minutes. We'll stop on our way home." He hung up, banging the receiver.

I sighed and postponed a previously scheduled appointment.

Forty minutes later Mr. and Mrs. Carson were seated in my office. Both were tall, well-dressed and appeared to be in their early thirties. Under different circumstances they would have made an attractive couple, but the man's taut, white face seemed at odds with his meticulously groomed blond hair, expensive jacket and silk tie. By the same token, the trim navy suit, color coordinated paisley blouse and matching shoes did not belong on such a silent, drooping woman. I had greeted the Carsons, offered coffee, which had been declined, and now we sat unspeaking. I glanced from one to the other expectantly. Jim Carson folded his arms across his chest and stared over my head with cold, belligerent eyes. Mrs. Carson drooped in a corner chair like a pale, fading blossom. I had noticed how slowly she walked, trailing behind her husband as he strode down the corridor to my office, and I wondered if she was still suffering from post-birth discomfort that made walking painful. Thinking of the long trek from the parking lot to my office I felt anger at Mr. Carson for forcing this ordeal upon her.

Carson finally broke the silence, addressing his wife. "You said you wanted to talk to her, so talk!"

Mary Carson lifted her head and brushed back a lock of dark hair. A pair of deep brown eyes bore into mine, but she remained silent.

"Where's the baby?" I prompted. "Still at the hospital?"

She nodded.

"Is anything wrong? Was the baby premature?"

"Oh, no, she's fine. The doctor said she's in perfect health ..." Mary Carson bit her lip and glanced at her husband. He was frowning, staring into space. Her dark eyes sought mine again.

"Would you like to keep your baby?"

"Yes." Mary bent her head. A tear fell on her tightly clenched hands. "That's why I wanted to talk to you ... to find out more about her condition ... perhaps it isn't that hopeless ... perhaps I could manage to take care of her ... "

"No way!" Carson interrupted brusquely. "I spoke to the hospital social worker before we came. It's all arranged."

"She ... she suggested we put the baby in a foster home." Mary whispered.

I nodded, agreeing that a temporary placement might be the best decision for the present. A brief separation would give them a chance to come to terms with their sorrow and to learn more about the potential of children with Down syndrome. I tried to explain how an infant program would benefit their little daughter, but Mr. Carson cut me off.

"What you say may be true, and it may work for some people, but not for us. My wife has a responsible position with an insurance company, she doesn't have time to fuss with these special programs, and as far as I'm concerned a mongoloid is just so many pounds of raw meat!"

Grief, frustration, despair can be expressed in many ways, and over the years I met scores of angry parents, but I had yet to hear a father reject his child with such shocking vehemence.

I turned to the mother, trying to diffuse this terrible moment.

"Does the baby have a name?"

Carson shifted impatiently, but before he could speak, Mary's magnificent eyes flashed with sudden defiance.

"Her name is Margaret. Maggie, after my mother."

Without another word they rose and left my office. Mary Carson walked rapidly, a few paces ahead of her husband, her back straight, her head held high. What would she do with this seemingly newly found strength, I wondered, divorce Jim Carson?

I never heard from Jim nor Mary Carson again. I don't know if their marriage survived his betrayal, nor whether they ever had another child. Three weeks later, however, I met Maggie and her foster mother, Betty Daniels.

Maggie was now the legal ward of the State and eligible for adoption. For the present, however, until an adoptive family could be found, she had been placed in foster care. On her case worker's recommendation, Mrs. Daniels enrolled Maggie in the Infant Program and I met the pair on their initial visit to the Unit. Maggie's surrogate mom was in her mid twenties, and like Maggie's biological mother, she was a tall, dark-haired woman. Unlike Mary Carson, however, who was thin as a model, Betty was as cozy as a feather bed: all curves and softness — breasts like twin mounds of rising dough, plump arms and a round, smiling face. She entered my office carrying Maggie, lovingly cradled against her ample shoulder and yielding bosom. My spirits soared in a sudden surge of happiness.

What a fortuitous placement for an unwanted, abandoned baby, I thought, as Mrs. Daniels sat down, and holding Maggie on her lap, gently turned back the fluffy pink blanket that had been hiding the baby's face. Maggie was asleep. A thick fringe of long, black lashes rimmed the curve of her chubby cheeks. A rosy mouth pouted in sleep and wisps of black hair encircled her head in a halo.

"Oh, what a beautiful baby!"

"Yes," Betty flushed with pride and pleasure. "Notice her coloring, just like mine. You'd think she was my own baby! My very own ... in fact ... I already think of her as our own ... she's so sweet!"

The passing months proved that I had not been mistaken in my estimate of Betty Daniels nor in the kind of home I sensed that she and her husband would be able to give Maggie. I had yet to meet Bob Daniels, but from what Betty told me I judged that he was an equally loving foster parent. Meanwhile Maggie thrived, making rapid gains in her development. By the time she entered the Toddler Program at eighteen months Maggie was already walking and beginning to repeat one or two words. Since children with Down syndrome are generally delayed in walking and speaking, Maggie's achievements were welcomed as accelerated development. On the whole Maggie was a cheerful, self-sufficient child who interacted happily with her classmates and delighted her teachers.

Another year went by and as I observed Betty's unchanging warmth towards Maggie, and Maggie's complete confidence in Betty's love and approval, I became convinced that it was only a matter of time before the Daniels would take the final step and make Maggie their legally adopted daughter.

Then one day Betty requested a conference with me. As soon as she seated herself in my office I noticed that she appeared troubled and yet, at the same time, her face glowed with a new inner radiance. For once Betty seemed reluctant to speak. I broke the silence.

"Is anything wrong, Betty?"

"Well, yes, and no. Oh, Val!" She caught my hand suddenly. "The most remarkable thing has happened. I'm going to have a baby!"

"How wonderful! I'm so happy for you!"

Sharing her joy, I felt tears spring to my eyes. I knew how desperately Betty and Bob had yearned to have a child. They had already been married five years when they took Maggie into their home. Undoubtedly the little girl filled a void in their lives, but they had not been able to resign themselves to Betty's inexplicable childlessness.

"You're sure?" I persisted.

"Oh, yes. I'm more than three months along, and the doctor assures me that all should go well." She smiled but her eyes still looked troubled.

"So, what's bothering you, Betty?"

Her voice was low. "Maggie."

Then she hurried on, as if fearing I would prevent her from saying what she had to tell me. "I ... Bob ... we can't keep her. She's a darling little girl ... we love her, we really do ... you know that ... but now, now that I'm going to have my own baby ... I ... I don't want to be distracted ... This is such a special time for Bob and me ... we have waited and hoped for so long ... it's silly, I know, and probably terribly unfair ... but ... but I almost resent Maggie now, as if she's already taking me away from my baby ... and later, after the baby comes ... I'm afraid it will be worse ... "

Tears glittered in her eyes.

"I suppose you think I'm terrible for feeling this way."

"Not at all," I assured her. "I understand how you feel, and I respect your honesty."

"I've already spoken to my social worker," Betty continued. "They have a client who would like to adopt Maggie. Her name is Hannah Buhler, she's a widow, from Holland. She used to be a teacher."

In the past only married couples were allowed to adopt children, but the laws had become more flexible, especially in the case of a handicapped child, so I didn't question the possibility of a single woman adopting Maggie. Still the news hit me like a blow to the diaphragm. Poor little Maggie, I thought clutching my middle. My lips felt stiff, but I forced myself to speak calmly, to keep my expression neutrally pleasant.

"I hope I can meet Mrs. Buhler," I said.

"Of course you will," Betty promised, explaining that Mrs. Buhler lived in the area and that Maggie would continue attending classes at the Unit. From a telephone conversation with Mrs. Buhler, Betty was confident that Maggie would find a happy, permanent home.

Betty left the building smiling, relieved, no doubt, that her distressing news had been accepted, and I had smiled in return. Despite my disappointment and misgivings, as far as Maggie was concerned, I was sincerely glad for Betty and Bob Daniels. They had been conscientious and loving parents to Maggie during the crucial formative months of her babyhood, and I could understand their desire to ready themselves for the long awaited birth of their own child, unburdened by the undeniable and sometimes excessive demands of a child with special needs, even a child as healthy, and appealing as Maggie. Still as I contemplated Maggie's future an oppressive pall settled over me. Later when Mrs. Buhler telephoned me and in her Dutch-accented English requested permission to visit Maggie's classroom, I scolded myself for my depression and tried to view the situation more optimistically. After all, I wasn't ready to adopt the child myself, I reasoned, so why should I prejudge someone who was ready to commit herself to Maggie's future and who was apparently in agreement with our educational goals for Maggie and the other children in the program?

Hannah Buhler came the following Monday. As I guided her into the observation booth I asked her if she would be able to recognize Maggie.

"Yah, I see pictures," she replied, nodding as she caught sight of Maggie through the one-way glass. Maggie was in the housekeeping area, bustling about, a busy little homemaker, setting the table with toy dishes, and feeding imaginary cereal to a doll in a doll-sized high chair. The mannerisms and activity reminded me of Betty Daniels, smiling I glanced at my companion. Her face was set, almost stern, but when I spoke to her she nodded.

"Yah, good."

When a thin smile touched her pale lips I tried to feel encouraged.

As we observed I explained that the toddler and preschool classes met for two hours four days a week. The kindergarten pupils attended school five days for two and a half hours per day. Each class was staffed by a head teacher who had a Master's degree in Early Childhood Special Education and her assistant, usually a university student majoring in education. Additionally, I reminded Mrs. Buhler, each parent, father, mother, or prime caregiver (as in the case of working or single parents) participated in the classroom one day a week. This arrangement benefited the program by increasing the pupil-adult ratio resulting in more individualized attention and better supervision. The main purpose of this requirement, however, was to continue the parent involvement that began at the infant level, to further the parents' training in specific instructional procedures and to maintain an ongoing dialogue between school and home. My job, as coordinator was to supervise the overall program, provide in-service staff training and to conference parents. Having said all this, I invited Mrs. Buhler into the classroom.

The children, absorbed in their various activities, scarcely glanced in our direction as we made our way to two small chairs on the other side of the room. At five feet and two inches, I had no trouble sitting on the low stool, but Mrs. Buhler who towered six or seven inches above me, looked like a stork perching on a chicken roost. I suggested a higher chair, but she refused my offer.

As the morning progressed I made soft-voiced comments, calling her attention to Maggie, emphasizing the child's attention span, her compliance with teacher directions, her willingness to attempt difficult tasks and her friendly responses to other children. The woman beside me kept nodding and saying, "Yah, yah," offering nothing in return. At one point Penny, the head teacher, came up to speak to us. Shorter than I, Penny was a tiny wren of a girl, with a sharp, elfin face and bones that seemed as fragile as a bird's. She was a wonderful teacher, however, dedicated, creative, loving and gentle with the children. She was also fiercely loyal and ready to battle anyone and anything that might threaten their welfare. Penny smiled politely and gave Mrs. Buhler the classroom schedule and several other pieces of informational material. Despite the smile there was a hard glint in Penny's eyes and I sensed that she did not approve of Maggie's future adoptive parent.

Mrs. Buhler accepted the papers and gave one of her nods. "I teacher. I know already." She folded the papers in half and jammed them into her purse.

Then it was music time, the last activity of the day. The children and the adults sat in a circle on the rug. Penny played the piano. Everyone sang, clapped hands, banged on drums and shook bells. It was a noisy, exuberant and utterly charming performance. To my dismay, Mrs Buhler sat with her head down, boney hands cupped over her ears.

As the last song was sung, mothers, who had remained at home that day, began appearing in the doorway to take their little sons and daughters home. At this point Maggie approached our chairs. Betty, I knew, made all of Maggie's clothes, and this morning as always, Maggie looked as if she had stepped out of a little girls' fashion magazine. She wore a white blouse with puffed, laced-edged sleeves and a ruffled red pinafore over a short plaid skirt. Her glossy black hair, curling around plump, rosy cheeks was pinned back with twin red barrettes. Her chubby legs were clad in white knee-high socks and shiny black Mary Janes.[3] Maggie was such a healthy, cuddlesome child, I longed to hold her on my lap.

"Hi," said Maggie.

"Hi," I replied.

Hannah Buhler folded long arms over a flat chest and leaned forward, slightly. "Mama," she said. Maggie's face brightened and she pointed to the door where the entering mothers had gathered. "Ma-ma," she echoed.

"No." Mrs. Buhler pointed to herself. "I, Mama," she repeated sternly.

Maggie looked confused, then Betty Daniels appeared in the doorway, and Maggie toddled off joyfully to meet her.

Mrs. Buhler looked at me disapprovingly. "Margarete, not talk?"

"Maggie?"

"Yah, I call Margarete, not Maggie. Margarete proper name. She not talk?"

"You heard her, she says a few words. Children with Down syndrome rarely speak fluently at this age, even older children have difficulties, but she is learning.[4] You do understand that Maggie ... ah ... Margarete was born with Down syndrome? Down syndrome, you understand?"

"Yah, yah, I know. Mongoloid ... I make it go away!"

I stared at her aghast. *What was she talking about, how could she possibly make Maggie's genetic condition go away?* Before I could reply or protest, Hannah Buhler pushed her self up from the little chair and followed Maggie and Betty out the door.

Penny clutched my arm. "We can't let that woman take Maggie," she hissed.

"I know. I'm calling the social worker right away."

"You must reconsider this placement!" I insisted, listing all the reasons why I thought Mrs. Buhler would not make a good mother for Maggie.

"She has excellent references," the social worker, Mrs. Randall, countered. "A nice home, very well kept, a good income. Her late husband left Mrs. Buhler well situated. Few single parents have these advantages, and she's most anxious to adopt Maggie. Most adoptive parents want infants. It isn't often that we find a perspective parent for a three-year-old handicapped child, especially at such a short notice. Do you realize how many children we have on our waiting list, all in need of placement, especially permanent homes? Surely you know that the demand for foster care and adoption far exceeds what is available." Mrs. Randall sounded very cross with me.

"Yes, I know, I know ... but Mrs. Buhler seems so cold."

"I didn't find her so. Reserved, perhaps, maybe even shy, but cold, oh, no, you misjudge her."

"How old is Mrs. Buhler?"

"Forty-seven. A good age, mature enough to be reliable, and still young enough to care for a small child."

I was still indignant.

"What she said when she called Maggie a mongoloid is absolutely ridiculous! Down syndrome is a chromosomal abnormality. How can she make it go away?"

"Oh, you misunderstood her. Mrs. Randall spoke soothingly as she would to an unreasonable client. Besides," she concluded, "Bob and Betty Daniels are going on a vacation. They're flying to Hawaii this coming Friday. So what can we do?"

Finally, sensing my distress, Mrs. Randall reminded me that every adoption begins with a trial period. Nothing would be finalized for at least six months, maybe a year. And, yes, definitely, Maggie would continue coming to school. That was the agreement. Hannah would participate in the classroom with the rest of the mothers. We would come to know her. Everything would work out for the best, and if not, well, time was on our side.

Acquiescing reluctantly, I said good-bye and went in search of Penny.

"I don't care!" stormed Penny, after I had related my conversation with Mrs. Randall. "Maybe that woman is not as bad as she seems, but believe me I'm going to watch her like a ferret!"

I patted Penny on the shoulder. "I know you will."

The next three days passed swiftly, uneventfully and suddenly it was Thursday, the last school day for the toddler class. At the end of that morning's session, instead of going home with Betty Daniels, Maggie left for a new life with Hannah Buhler.

I spent an anxious weekend worrying about Maggie. Monday morning found me hurrying to the toddler classroom. My eyes swept over the children gathered in a circle for group time. Karl, the student teacher, was leading them in a song.

"Where is Johnny, where is Johnny?" he sang.

"Here!" called out a blond three-year-old, Maggie's special friend.

But where was Maggie? I caught Penny's eye. She shook her head.

"Where is she?" I demanded, following Penny to the far side of the room.

"Sick. Mrs. Buhler telephoned this morning."

"What's wrong?"

Penny looked doubtful. "Just a cold, according to Mrs. B."

"Oh, dear. Did she say anything else? How are they getting along?"

"Fine, I guess," Penny responded gloomily.

"Maggie never gets a cold," I persisted.

"I know. This will be the first time she's been absent this year."

We both knew that children with Down syndrome are especially susceptible to colds and upper respiratory infections so we had come to accept some absenteeism as inevitable. This was different. Maggie, the one exception, enjoyed consistently good health. This change in her physical well-being troubled us.

"I suppose this is to be expected. Stress, new surroundings, a new routine, homesickness ..."

Penny looked ready to cry. "Enough to make anyone sick. Enough to make me sick!"

"Well, at least Mrs. Buhler telephoned."

Penny continued to look unhappy. "Yeah, big deal."

"Make a note of this. Let's keep a record for the time being."

"I'll start a log right away," Penny agreed. "I'll keep track of everything that happens."

I returned to my office fighting the urge to telephone Mrs. Buhler, to jump into my car and drive over to visit Maggie. Yet I knew that I had to be tactful, such a move might only antagonize Mrs. Buhler, for Maggie's sake I had to win the woman's confidence.

Ten days passed before we saw Maggie again, and when we did we were shocked to find her standing forlornly in the hall leading to the classroom. At age four the children were transported to school on regular school buses, but until that time each parent was responsible for delivering her child directly into the classroom. In leaving Maggie to wander about unattended her new mother broke a cardinal rule. But we were even more shocked by Maggie's appearance and behavior. In place of the sparkling, rosy-faced youngster we saw a hollow eyed, pathetic little waif who trembled and shrunk back when approached.

Sensing that Maggie was unaccountably intimidated by her attention, Penny drew back and told everyone else to do the same. Left alone, Maggie crept to the housekeeping area, then finding her favorite doll, she huddled in a corner, holding the doll and sucking her thumb. Troubled by what had happened, Penny phoned the school nurse, but Miss Perkins couldn't come right away. A five year-old boy in one of the other classes fell on his way to school, skinning his knee. The nurse said that she would check on Maggie as soon as she finished attending to his wound. However, before Miss Perkins could come, Maggie wet her pants and burst into whimpering sobs.

As every mother and teacher of young children knows, wet pants and soiled diapers are a fact of life, and such incidents are handled philosophically. Maggie, however, had been toilet trained since she was two and a half and there hadn't been a single accident for the past five or six months. So this lapse was another indication that Maggie might be much sicker than we had assumed or that something else was seriously wrong.

I, of course, knew nothing of this until my phone rang and Penny's voice shrieked in my ear.

"That woman is beating Maggie! There are two great big purple bruises on her bottom! You can even see the full imprint of a hand!"

"I'm coming!" I shouted and leaped up from my desk.

I found the classroom in an uproar. The school social worker and the nurse were already there, and Penny, arming herself for warfare was taking Poloroid pictures of the incriminating bruises. Children, bewildered by the commotion, milled about, mothers crowded together, buzzing with indignation. Maggie lay on the changing table sobbing in shuddering little gasps.

Gradually order was restored. A spare pair of dry panties replaced Maggie's wet one, and Alice Nyman, blond Johnny's mother, who happened to be working in the classroom that day offered to comfort Maggie. Alice Nyman and Betty Daniels were friends and Johnny and Maggie frequently played together after school.

"Come, Maggie, I'll read you a story," she said reaching for the distressed little girl, and Maggie, recognizing a friend, clung to Mrs. Nyman with the fierceness of a bear cub clinging to a tree top. Soon Alice Nyman was sitting on a rug with Maggie on her lap and Johnny by her side, reading a picture book to the two children.

When our social worker left to telephone Mrs. Randall at the adoption agency, the nurse reported that she had weighed and measured Maggie and found that the child had lost three and a half pounds and appeared undernourished and dehydrated.

"Maggie has either been seriously ill or she has been denied food," Miss Perkins concluded.

"She's not going back to that woman!" Penny clenched her fists and glared at me defiantly.

"Not for a minute," I agreed, thinking of all that would have to be done, the people that I might have to involve and preparing to take Maggie home with me, if necessary. Then to my utmost relief and amazement the whole matter resolved itself with unbelievable speed and simplicity.

In speaking to Mrs. Randall, our school social worker learned that Hannah Buhler had already been in contact with the agency. Mrs. Buhler, it turned out, had a long list of complaints. She had been told, Buhler grumbled, that Maggie was toilet trained, but on the very first night the child had wet her bed.

"I spank!" declared Mrs. Buhler indignantly, "I say, 'wet bed, no breakfast!' She still wet bed. I take away drink, milk, water, bed wet! I spank hard, no good. She pee on floor! Bad girl, stubborn! I don't want!"[5]

When Mrs Randall replied that Maggie would be removed from her home immediately, Mrs. Buhler said: "Good. I bring things. Leave at school."

Now we had to decide what to do about Maggie.

"I can take her home with me," I said.

"No, I will," said Penny.

"I will," countered Mrs. Nyman. "I'll take her home with me today, and I'm going to keep her. My husband and I have been talking about Maggie. She and Johnny are such good friends we want to adopt her. We wanted to do this from the very beginning, but everything happened so fast, we never had a chance to say anything."

Hannah Buhler left Maggie's belongings at the front office of the Unit without anyone of us ever seeing her again. Maggie went home with Mrs. Nyman and Johnny and has been a part of that warm, loving family ever since.

In retrospect I would like to say that I don't believe that Mrs. Buhler was a vicious or deliberately cruel person. What she did to Maggie was done out of ignorance and misguided expectations. As a recently widowed, middle-aged, childless woman she was undoubtedly lonely, and so perhaps fantasized that a little girl would fill this emptiness. She behaved, in fact, in the manner of someone who decides to obtain a pet dog or cat. Although it must be emphasized the pets also deserve caring, responsible owners who understand an animal's basic needs. This was Mrs. Buhler's problem. She may have been a teacher, but obviously she knew nothing about the development or the emotional and physical needs of young children.

This incident underscores the enormous responsibility that is placed upon those who supervise the placement of children in foster care and adoptive homes. Most of the time these placements are successful and children are given surrogate parents who, like, Bob and Betty Daniels, wholeheartedly provide loving homes for disadvantaged youngsters. However, none of us is infallible, and occasionally a child is placed inappropriately or allowed to remain in an abusive home. Then it is the moral duty of teachers and other persons who might become aware of a child's neglect or abuse to become that child's advocate and to be as ready to battle for that child's welfare as Penny had been to defend Maggie.

Chapter Two
Tommy and How it All Began

Whenever I'm asked what prompted me to devote my life to working with developmentally delayed children, I immediately think of Tommy and something that happened in the spring of 1958. At that time I was working as a Family Life instructor for the Seattle Public Schools. My job was to act as adviser to community based parent cooperative preschools. I gave help and training to nursery school teachers, conducted meetings and held child development classes for the parents. It was also my responsibility to serve as a liaison between the Family Life parent education program and the preschools, making sure that the standards for a superior preschool program were consistently maintained. At this point in my life I had a B.A. degree from the University of Washington and considerable additional training in early childhood education, but I had yet to pursue graduate degrees in special education. The children in the preschools that I supervised showed typical development.

The five preschools that I visited weekly were located in Bellevue, a suburban community on the east side of Lake Washington, in Seattle. Thirty-one years ago, Bellevue was yet to become the traffic congested, burgeoning city that it is today with its soaring office buildings, glittering boutiques, fashionable restaurants and spacious shopping malls. Yet, even in 1958, anticipating the completion of a second floating bridge across Lake Washington, destined to provide an easy commute to Seattle, affluent couples were beginning to throng to expansive new developments to live in gracious homes on large, landscaped lots. Still, despite this influx of new residents, Bellevue, at that time, was mainly an area of farms, undeveloped land and forests thick with massive Douglas firs, graceful hemlocks and ancient cedars. In the spring dogwoods dotted this dark greenery with bursts of white, four-petalled blossoms. Maples and alders swung pollen-yellowed catkins in the breeze. In October the woodlands became a vast tapestry against whose emerald background autumn colored trees wove their gold and scarlet skeins.

Situated between two huge bodies of water, twenty-two mile long Lake Washington on the west and Lake Sammamish to the east, Bellevue lies like a polished jade stone set between two luminous sapphires. Across Lake Sammamish timbered foothills undulate, ascending eastward to erupt in the granite grandeur of the Cascade range. These majestic mountains traverse the state from north to south like a Great Wall of China. To the west of Lake Washington, beyond Puget Sound, the Olympic mountains and the jagged snow-capped peaks of Mount Olympus dominate the horizon.

My husband, Nick, our three children and I moved to Bellevue in 1953, long before builders bulldozed their first plot of raw land. Our thirteen-year-old, Cathy, wanted a horse. The two boys, Mike, eight, and Alex, five, needed space to run and play. Nick and I wanted the peace of country living with room for a horse, a German Shephard and a cat. We found and purchased an abandoned schoolhouse situated on seven acres of land. The old Phantom Lake school (actual name) was a two-storied building with a single classroom. Within a year we successfully converted the deserted old structure into a comfortable three-bedroom home with a large basement and family room.

The majority of the women who enrolled their children in the preschools which I supervised, lived in much grander houses than our remodeled dwelling. They belonged, as I said, to the upwardly mobile, affluent population that was finding its way to the beautiful Eastside. The young women wore cashmere sweaters and cultured pearls. They drove powerful new cars. This was the baby boom era. Bright, healthy, handsome, neatly-dressed youngsters filled the cooperative preschools.

Although it was my responsibility to guide the children's program, the preschools were autonomous. The schools belonged to the parents. Parents paid the rent, the teacher's salary and all other expenses. They had their own board of elected officers, and their own bylaws. My salary, on the other hand, was paid by the Seattle Public Schools, and I was not a voting member of the preschools. I could advise, instruct, recommend, but I could not dictate. I enjoyed my work and my relationship with the groups under my care had always been warm and mutually supportive. Then at the beginning of Spring quarter in 1958, Sylvia Morvick enrolled her son, Tommy.

Sylvia did not live in a fashionable home in an exclusive area. She did not drive a Thunderbird or a Mercedes, nor did she wear cashmeres and pearls. The Morvicks lived in the backwoods of Bellevue on a small semi-cleared tract of land in an crumbling old farm house. Their car was a rust-corroded Chevy pickup. Sylvia's shapeless cotton dress came from a catalogue, her nylons were a man's socks rolled down around her ankles and her alligator pumps were a pair of scuffed, runover loafers. Thin, silent and withdrawn, with drooping shoulders, hair that was limp and colorless as winter's beaten grass and pale gray eyes which peered myopically through steel-framed glasses that kept slipping to the end of her red-tipped nose, poor Sylvia was as dull and faded as her $4.97 dress. Among her energetic, self-assured peers, she was a bedraggled sparrow surrounded by a flock of brilliant parakeets. Worse yet, her newly enrolled little boy, Tommy, was retarded.

Physically Tommy appeared as normal as any other four-year-old. He was tall for his age, sturdy and well coordinated, but Tommy did not speak, not a single word.

Tommy screeched, Tommy screamed, Tommy threw tantrums. He tore about the classroom like a tornado. He grabbed, he threw, he snatched displays off the bulletin board, he kicked, he shoved, he attacked the other children and he bit. He had a voracious appetite and his manners were atrocious.

The Mountain View Preschool met in the afternoon. Bringing their sandwiches, the children and mothers arrived at noon to sit down to a sociable lunch before beginning the daily activities. The spring term had been in operation for three days and Tommy had been in attendance for as many days, when I arrived for my scheduled visit on the fourth day. I came, anxious to meet Tommy and his mother. Since the first day of the new term I had been hearing a great deal about Tommy. Every afternoon and evening I received phone calls from indignant mothers reporting on Tommy's misdeeds.

"That child is a monster!" they told me.

"He hit Susie with a block!"

"He's dangerous. He pushed Peter off the slide."

"He bit Amy and Jason. Yesterday he tried to bite the teacher!"

"What about his mother?" I asked. "What does Mrs. Morvick do while all of this is going on?"

I knew that I could expect Sylvia to be present because all newly enrolled mothers were required to remain with their children for the first few days. Later the mothers were scheduled to work only one day a week, following the same plan that I adapted to the program for children with Down syndrome at the Experimental Education Unit. In answer to my questions, the women were equally critical of Sylvia.

"Oh, she's a mess!" a mother snapped.

"I suppose she tries," another conceded. "She tries to stop him, but he's too quick."

"Half the time she doesn't know any better, from the looks of her," they sneered.

I arrived at lunch time, just as the group gathered around a large, low table. Pulling over a preschool-sized chair, I sat down next to Sylvia. Grace was said, all the seated children began decorously unwrapping their peanut butter and jelly sandwiches, all except Tommy. Tommy was squirming and fussing, struggling with his mother who was trying to restrain him, as he fought to escape.

"He doesn't want to sit!" she gasped forcing a leg back under the table. "He never sits at home, I cannot get him to sit down to eat!"

I stood up and put restraining hands on Tommy's shoulders. He began to screech. In desperation Sylvia hurriedly shelled a hard-boiled egg and gave it to Tommy. Tommy grabbed the egg and crammed the whole thing in his mouth. Choking on this huge mouthful Tommy began to cough, sputtering egg bits all over the table. As mothers looked on with revulsion, Tommy sprang up from the table, and tearing across the room knocked down an elaborate block building that another boy had laboriously constructed the previous afternoon and which the teacher had promised to save. As the blocks clattered to the floor, Tommy shrieked with delight dribbling more egg down his chin.

After seeing Tommy in action, and after hearing complaints all week I was not surprised by a summons from the president of the preschool to attend an emergency meeting — "of the most vital importance" — that evening. When I appeared at the home where the meeting was held I found that the entire membership, including the teacher, was present. Only Sylvia Morvick was noticeably absent. She had not been invited. As I suspected the purpose of the meeting was to air grievances against Tommy and to vote him and his mother out of the group. Before the vote was taken, however, I made an eloquent plea on their behalf.

The purpose of the preschools, I argued, was to teach parents techniques of child management and to help children learn appropriate social behaviors. I called on the teacher and the mothers to help Sylvia and Tommy. I outlined a set of rules and limits for Tommy, suggesting strategies for coping with his distressing behaviors. I was gratified when finally the teacher and the majority of the women supported me. The decision was made to allow Tommy to remain for two more weeks on a trial basis. I told the group that I would reschedule my visits to the other four preschools under my care and that I would come to Mountain View every day during this trial period in order to keep an eye on Tommy and to help the teacher inaugurate the outlined strategies.

The meeting had been held on Thursday, the last school day for the week. Over the weekend I telephoned Sylvia, and told her as gently as I could that in order to benefit from the preschool experience, Tommy would have to learn to follow directions and comply with class rules. Although Sylvia had little to say, she appeared to welcome my suggestions. In any case, on the following Monday the afternoon session began auspiciously. In accordance with our plan Sylvia didn't bring Tommy to school until after lunch. When she did arrive, Sylvia appeared more relaxed, and Tommy, with remnants of a sandwich on his face, also appeared to be in a more tractable mood.

Nevertheless, as the day progressed, I kept a fixed eye on Tommy, alert as a bodyguard to any signs of trouble. Twice, by intervening quickly, I was able to avert disaster, once when Tommy seemed on the verge of shoving a younger child to the floor and another time when he snatched a hammer from the woodworking bench and aimed to hurl it through the window.

When it was time for the children to go outside to play, the teacher asked me to remain inside with Stephen, a docile redheaded little boy, who was recovering from a cold and who was not yet well enough for vigorous outdoor play. I readily agreed and invited Tommy and his mother to stay with me.

"This will be a good opportunity for Stephen and Tommy to get acquainted," I told the teacher, Miss Lois.

Sylvia joined me as I led the two boys to the block corner and seated them on the floor beside me. Stephen immediately began laying one block on top of the other, building a tower. Picking up a block, I placed it in Tommy's hand, showing him how he too could add blocks to Stephen's structure. Each time Stephen placed a block, I handed one to Tommy and guided his hand until the piece of wood had been placed correctly. As we worked I kept up a stream of encouragement.

"Good for you, Tommy. That's the way to do it. Here's another block. You and Stephen are building a big tower."

Yet all the time I remained tensely watchful, determined to prevent any movement that Tommy might make toward hitting Stephen, throwing a block or knocking over the building. Minutes passed, Tommy and Stephen continued their play. It even seemed to me that Tommy was beginning to anticipate my actions, reaching for a block before I had actually dropped it in his hand. Sylvia, who had been sitting silently on my right, said something. I turned my head. A piercing cry shattered the quietness of the room. In the split second that I had looked away, Tommy sunk his teeth into Stephen's arm. Before I could do anything Sylvia grabbed Tommy's arm and bit him in return, drawing blood. As Tommy howled, Sylvia clutched her head and fell to the floor in a screaming hysterical fit.

On hearing the terrible shrieks the teacher, mothers and children came running into the room, and there I was, their esteemed instructor, the "expert," trying to deal with two wailing boys and a sobbing, incoherent woman. Had I been a sheriff in a Western movie, I would have turned in my badge! Then as the agitated mothers and children crowded around us, Sylvia scrambled to her feet, snatched up Tommy and fled from the room. I handed Stephen to Miss Lois and ran after her.

Tommy was already in the truck, using his teeth to open a package of chocolate cookies. Sylvia was in the driver's seat, ready to slam the door.

I laid a hand on her arm. "Sylvia, wait."

She jerked away. 'I'm not going back!"

"I know."

"They don't like Tommy!" She began polishing her tear-stained glasses with the hem of her dress.

"It's not that they don't like Tommy. It's just ... well ... that Tommy has ... ah ... problems."

She looked at me dully and I wondered fleetingly if Sylvia herself might not be slightly retarded, or was she simply so beaten down by frustration, a sense of helplessness, and life in general, that she gave that impression. In fact, if her earlier hysteria was any indication, she might well be on the verge of an emotional collapse.

"Tommy may not be ready for this particular preschool," I continued. "It may be too stimulating for him, too exciting."

Sylvia was nodding her head slightly, listening to me.

"Did it ever occur to you that Tommy might be a little ... " I hesitated, but it had to be said, *"retarded?"*

She looked at me, her gray eyes strangely enlarged, like pebbles under water.

"I ... I thought he was ... just ... you know, wild."

"That's what I mean. It isn't normal for a child to be so wild," I told her.

Sylvia didn't answer.

"How do you manage at home?" I asked.

"He stays in the crib."

"All the time!"

"Most of the time."

"What does he do, doesn't he try to get out?"

"No, he just jumps up and down on the bed. He's worn out three mattresses already."

"Doesn't he have any toys?"

"He breaks them." For the second time her tear-brimmed eyes met mine. "Why is he like that? Wild, I mean?"

I shook my head sadly. 'I don't know."

I didn't add that Tommy was the first child with such disruptive behaviors that I had ever encountered in the eight years that I had worked in the Family Life Program, nor could I admit that I knew absolutely nothing about mental retardation, nothing about the possible causes of such abnormal behavior nor what could be done to help these children. Remembering Tommy,

I now suspect that he was brain damaged, possibly autistic, and perhaps deaf. In any case, knowing what I know now, I should have referred Tommy to a neurologist for a brain scan, to an audiologist for a hearing test and to a psychologist for an evaluation of his intelligence. It occurs to me now that Tommy may have had normal or near normal intelligence. Brain damage and a severe hearing loss could certainly account for Tommy's aggressive hyperactivity and lack of speech.

To this day I regret that due to my total ignorance I was unable to give Tommy and his mother all the help that they needed. Nevertheless, even then, I knew enough to realize that I couldn't allow Tommy to return to the isolation of his crib. Such deprivation could only lead to complete psychosis, and was, undoubtedly, already aggravating Tommy's wildness and antisocial tendencies. Tommy needed to learn how to handle toys and materials appropriately. He needed to be shown how to interact with other children. He needed many positive, enriching experiences. No wonder he behaved like a wild animal in school. In reality his crib was no better than a cage.

Sylvia was not an abusive mother. Her desperate attack on Tommy when she bit him, was, I fully believe, a one-time occurrence, brought on by unbearable frustration and an all-consuming need to make Tommy acceptable to the group. There was no evidence of previous abuse. Tommy was certainly well-nourished. His garments appeared to come from the Goodwill, but they were clean and apparently chosen with some care. There were no telltale bruises on his body. Still it was imperative to give Sylvia better ways of managing his uncontrollable behaviors. Sylvia was not abusive, but her method of dealing with Tommy by imprisoning him in his bed, did in fact constitute abuse. It was morally wrong and it was potentially dangerous. As Tommy grew older and became even more unmanageable, I could foresee terrible acts of violence as Sylvia's only recourse.

I glanced at Tommy. He was stuffing the last of the cookies into his mouth, spilling crumbs all over his shirt. Sylvia moistened a crumpled tissue with her lips and gently wiped his chocolate-smeared cheeks. Deep compassion for Tommy and his mother filled my heart. Again I laid a hand on her arm. This time she didn't draw away.

"I'm not giving up on Tommy," I told her. "He needs a group experience ... not a regular preschool, perhaps, but something ... I'll see what I can do. I'll phone you as soon as I have something definite."

I closed the cab door. Sylvia turned on the ignition. The motor sputtered, the truck shuddered, jerked, and rolled out of the parking lot. I watched, a plan forming in my mind. Within seconds an idea had taken root and flowered into a firm commitment. I would organize a parent cooperative preschool for children with special needs. And I did.

Chapter Three
Transition

The preschool for handicapped children began with six pupils including Tommy. The parents of this new group came in response to a notice that I placed in the local paper. Like the Morvicks, these families came from the outskirts of Bellevue, troubled, hard-working people of modest means. It would appear that affluent couples did not have retarded children, for none showed up at our first organizational meeting. More likely the developmentally delayed children of well-to-do families attended private schools.

As I welcomed the six families to our newly formed preschool it became obvious that such a small group of low-income parents could not afford to rent classroom space nor pay a teacher's salary. I made some inquiries, and the Faith Lutheran Church of Bellevue came to our aid by graciously donating the use of their kindergarten room, rent free, one day a week. We still needed a teacher, so I volunteered to lead the class on Friday mornings.

Since Tommy's original preschool, Mountain View, met in the afternoons, while the remaining four groups held morning sessions, I had, from the very beginning scheduled all my visits within a four-day period. This arrangement now left me free to take on the Handicapped Preschool on Fridays.

In view of my blatant inexperience it was undoubtedly audaciously conceited if not downright impertinent of me to bring these people together and offer a program for their children. Perhaps my actions can be justified on the grounds that there was nothing better. In 1958 public schools did not offer programs for so-called trainable retarded children. Children, who it was believed, could not benefit from an academic curriculum. As young adults these children might be placed in the sheltered workshops, meanwhile they were either institutionalized or kept at home, denied training and social contact with their peers.

This same policy applied to the severely profoundly handicapped population. These children were so severely impaired physically and mentally that many remained bedridden, scarcely aware of their environment, all their lives. A number of these children were blind as well as deaf. Because of their extreme helplessness and the heavy burden that their care placed on the family, the majority of these profoundly affected youngsters were institutionalized early in life. Nevertheless there were always some parents who bravely continued caring for their child at home. The Nielsons, who enrolled their little son Bernie in the preschool for handicapped children, were such parents.

Five-year-old Bernie could neither walk nor talk. He was a small child, with lank, almost white hair, a shrunken little face and enormous, cornflower blue eyes. His frail body was scarcely more than a skeleton wrapped in a thin layer of bluish white skin the color of diluted skimmed milk. His arms were like twigs, and his poor useless legs like withered branches, criss-crossed together in rigid immobility. Even sadder than Bernie's appearance was his cry. Bernie cried ceaselessly, a soft, keening, tearless whine, the endless moaning of someone in unbearable, unescapable pain. Rocking helped. So Bernie's mother held and rocked him, hour after hour.

When they came to school, I relieved her of this burden. Taking Bernie in my arms I danced him around the room. Round and round we went to a recording of Tchaikovsky's lilting *Waltz of the Flowers*. The dancing soothed Bernie and, as he grew quieter, something resembling a smile stretched his bloodless lips.

Among the remaining five pupils, Tommy was the youngest and the most retarded. The other boys ranged in age from six to twelve, and although they were all slow in their development, they were basically quiet, responsive children. There were no girls in the group. Statistics show that in the total population of mentally retarded individuals males outnumber females, so I was not surprised.

I ran a low-keyed, relaxed program. The children were kept busy with water, sand and dough play, crayons and easel paints. There was a story time and a social period when mothers and children sat down together for juice and crackers. There was a great deal of music; music for singing, marching and dancing.

Although the six mothers who brought their children every Friday morning took turns in helping me with the program, there were many opportunities for them to remain on the sidelines, to observe, to talk among themselves, freed, at least briefly, from the constant demands of their young. I was convinced that the mothers and children alike benefited from this respite. I also hoped that the women were learning new ways of coping with their children and of keeping them occupied.

All in all it appeared to be a happy experience for everyone. Even Tommy, although he still required close supervision, was no longer the terror that he had been at Mountain View. Once, however, he climbed, fully clothed, into the water table, and urinated into the water. Another time he jammed a roll of paper into the toilet bowl, and flushed the toilet. As the water cascaded to the floor, he hopped about shrieking with wild excitement. Nevertheless, compared to his previous behaviors, these were minor, isolated incidents.

The weeks slid uneventfully into June, and school was dismissed for the summer. The following September the preschool for handicapped children reopened with a flourish as a fully established program within the Family Life network. Classes resumed in a new location. We were now sharing space and equipment with one of the regular preschools under my supervision. A full enrollment of thirteen children generated enough tuition money for rent and a teacher's salary. The same teacher that taught the morning group of typical preschoolers agreed to teach the afternoon class for youngsters with disabilities. Both groups met three days a week.

The children in the reconvened preschool for the developmentally delayed ranged in age from three to eight. None was as severely involved as Bernie had been. Poor Bernie suffered a massive seizure, and died that summer. Tommy was also absent.

A few days after preschool had closed for the summer, I telephoned Sylvia. Although Sylvia told me that she was no longer keeping Tommy in the crib, having convinced her husband to fence in an outdoor area where he could play, I remained concerned about the boy. Sylvia, I believed, still needed a great deal of support and guidance.

"How's Tommy?" I asked.

"Gone," she said.

My hand clenched the receiver. "Gone! What do you mean? Where is he? What happened?"

"Tommy isn't here anymore."

Then in her lethargic, uncommunicative way, Sylvia told me that Tommy had been placed in a foster home with a woman who was experienced in caring for children like Tommy. I was stunned, almost too surprised to speak.

"How ... when ... ?" I sputtered.

"Paul's mom told me about that woman. Paul stays with her sometimes ... " her voice trailed off.

Paul was one of Tommy's former classmates. I had seen Sylvia talking to his mother. Sylvia amazed me. She appeared to be such an indecisive, ineffectual person, yet I knew that she could act with decisive, or was it desperate, suddenness. I tried to believe that Tommy would benefit from the placement, as I sensed the relief that this decision must have brought Sylvia. Still I wanted to know more, have more reassurance, I guess. In truth, perhaps I was disappointed, hurt, even, because Sylvia and her husband had acted without consulting me. Was Sylvia afraid that I would condemn her for what she wanted to do, or try to dissuade her? I hastened to reassure her. Parents of disabled children carry enough guilt, I had learned, without my adding to their burden.

"I'm sure you did the right thing," I told her. "Tommy is a difficult child. This foster mother may be able to help him."

"I ... I love Tommy ... I'm ... just so tired ... " her voice quivered on the verge of tears. "We ... didn't know what else to do."

Briefly, for an instant, as she had done on the day that she bit Tommy, Sylvia revealed herself, and then, just as quickly a veil of protective dullness dropped into place.

"I have to go ... I," she mumbled and hung up.

I never spoke to Sylvia again, and I don't know what became of Tommy, but I still remember him as I do many other children.

Chapter Four
State School

The next six years passed as swiftly as leaves flying in the wind. The preschool for children with disabilities continued to maintain a consistently high enrollment. Although I was no longer as intimately involved as I had been in the beginning, it remained under my supervision along with five preschools for typically developing children.

At home, my own children were growing up and leaving the nest. In 1960 our daughter Cathy married a doctoral student in the college of ceramic engineering. Three years later Mike became a freshman at the University of Washington, and our youngest son, Alex, started his first year at Newport High. Country living continued to be pleasant and fulfilling. Forsythias and rhododendrons bloomed in my garden. In the summer and fall we gathered cherries, plums and apples from our trees. Old dog, Rip, two cats and Peggy, our spirited but amiable Quarter horse added to the general sense of well-being. Like the sailboats on Lake Washington, my personal life and work skimmed along on an even keel. I should have been content, but I was growing progressively restless.

For one thing, I was dissatisfied with my role in the preschool for children with developmental delays. Although I visited the group faithfully and did my best to be supportive, I felt that my contacts were becoming increasingly superficial. Perhaps this was happening because as I learned more about mental retardation through reading and observation, I became increasingly aware of my inadequacies. I had lost the enthusiastic spontaneity with which I had organized our first preschool for disabled children. I cared for the children as deeply as ever, but I had come to realize that my present skills were not enough to give the children and their parents the kind of help they needed in order to make real progress.

Finally in 1963, the long-awaited Evergreen Point Bridge across Lake Washington was finished. Seattle and the University were now less than thirty minutes away. With my usual alacrity, I reached a decision.

"I'm going back to school," I announced to my family. "I'm going to get a Master's degree in Special Education."

Special education, as I was to learn, is a discipline as well as a service designed to serve children with special needs. These are the children who differ from the average, either physically or mentally, to such a degree that they are unable to make optimum progress in programs intended for the majority of school children. The gifted, as well as the mentally retarded, the blind, the deaf, the emotionally disturbed, the socially maladjusted as well as the physcially disabled and chronically health impaired are the exceptional children who require special education.

In order to serve such a wide spectrum of exceptionality, special education services consist of three elements. The first includes professional personnel, trained to serve specific categories of exceptionality. A teacher, for example, may be trained to work with the gifted or the blind, or as in my case, with the mentally retarded. The professional staff may also include teacher trainers, consultants, administrators, physiotherapists and speech therapists. The second component of special education is the curricular content. Classroom materials that are appropriate for typically developing children are likely to be too difficult for the disabled population and too elementary for the gifted pupils, so curriculum modification is necessary.

The third element of special education focuses on facilities. These include special building features such as ramps and toilet facilities. Special equipment such as group hearing aids, books with large print, magnifiers or braille, technical books for the gifted and low vocabulary-high-interest for the retarded are also a part of this third element.

At the moment that I had declared my intentions, I had but a vague idea of what special education entailed, but that did not trouble me. I had made my decision and the prospect excited me. I was ready to turn my back on what had come before and seek a new direction.

Birds were singing their early wake-up songs. The sun, cresting the Cascade mountains in a fiery arc lit up the sky with a golden-pink glow. It was June, 1964. A fine morning promised a perfect day. My husband, Nick, and the boys were still asleep when I stepped out of the house carrying my suitcase. Rip came out of his kennel, yawning and stretching, surprised, no doubt, by my early appearance. Tails aloft, the tips hooked like question marks, the cats bounded across the lawn to rub sinuous bodies against my legs. Peggy whinnied and trotted up to the pasture fence. Setting down my suitcase, I petted the animals and gave each

 Rainier State School

one a treat: a dog biscuit, cat kibbles, a pan of oats from the barn for Peggy. Five days would pass before I saw them again. I loaded my things into my fuchsia Rambler, a car that I purchased from a friend who was partial to that color, backed out of the carport, turned left, and headed south. *Graduate School, here I come!*

I was heading for the Rainier State School located in Buckley, Washington, a small farming community near the base of Mount Rainier, some eighty-five miles south of Bellevue. Earlier in the year I resigned from my Family Life job, to become effective at the end of the Spring term, and applied to Graduate School. As soon as I received word that I had been accepted, I signed up for my first two courses in special education: The Education of the Mentally Retarded and the Psychology of the Mentally Retarded. These were Summer quarter courses offered on location at the Rainier State School.

The classes would run for six weeks. Workshop participants had the option of commuting to and from the school or staying in a staff dormitory during the week. I decided to remain on campus, returning home for the weekends.

I drove towards my destination intoxicated with a wonderful sense of freedom and adventure. For the first time in twenty-five years of marriage, I was on my own. Married right out of college, I had never lived alone, never taken an extended trip by myself. Most of all, I had recently developed a consuming hunger to learn, to acquire new knowledge, and now I was on my way to a feast.

Rainier State School looked like a college campus. Stately two-storied white stucco buildings with red-tiled roofs, reminiscent of Spanish architecture, spread across expanses of brilliantly green grass. Here and there, scarcely noticeable among these fine buildings were a few barrack-like wooden buildings, intended, like the portables on school playgrounds, to accommodate a burgeoning population. Broad asphalt avenues crisscrossed the grounds. Trees, shrubs and occasional beds of marigolds, petunias and pansies bordered the sidewalks. Pastures and cultivated fields adjoined the campus on three sides.

I parked my car in front of the administration building and got out. There was no one in sight. The campus and the buildings seemed deserted, ominously quiet, like an enchanted kingdom. A flock of small white clouds grazing on Mount Rainier's crown, scattered and drifted across the sun. A chill passed over me. It was almost seven-thirty. Classes were scheduled to begin at eight. Where was everyone? Then, as I approached the administration hall, two more cars pulled into the driveway. Reassured, I entered the building and went in search of the registration desk.

Duly registered, armed with a map and key, my sense of excitement and adventure restored, I drove a short distance down the main avenue to the dormitory. It was a white stucco building, an exact replica of the imposing structures that dominated the campus. I reparked my car, loaded my arms with my belongings, mounted five brick steps and pulled open one side of the heavy double door. I stopped on the threshold, dismayed. A vast, dark, empty corridor, long and narrow as an alley stretched before me. Dark oak floors and equally dark, shoulder high wainscoting added to my sense of disorientation and claustrophobia. Then, as my eyes grew accustomed to the gloom, I discerned a series of numbered doors on either side of the hallway. Following the numbers I discovered my assigned room in the middle of a second corridor that joined the first to form a T. The second hall was shorter and not as somber as the first. Shafts of light from a barred window at either end lightened the gloom. I inserted the key into the lock and pushed on the solid oak door. It gave a protesting groan. I almost shuddered, wondering what would I find.

What I found was a small, pleasant room, spartan, but clean and bright. A large window overlooked a pasture. There were no bars. A desk, a chair, a chest of drawers, a cot with a white spread, a small closet and a bathroom with a tub provided everything that I might require. Wasting no time I unpacked, hung up my clothing, grabbed a notebook, extra pencils and a pen and hurried to my first class. It was almost eight o'clock.

Hurrying to my destination I noticed that the grounds were no longer deserted. A number of residents, mostly adolescents with Down syndrome were moving about doing yard work.

The class met in one of the low wooden buildings. Our main instructor was Dr. Barbra Etzel* from Western Washington University. She turned out to be an exceedingly charming woman, beautifully groomed with a becoming hairstyle, and a seemingly unlimited supply of elegant clothes. In fact I can't remember that she ever wore the same outfit more than once. Nevertheless her charm and elegance would have meant little to me had she not been an excellent teacher as well. Her lectures were as finely honed as her manicured nails, as carefully coordinated as her wardrobe. Precise and organized, her lectures retained the warmth and spontaneity, the genuine passion of a dedicated and inspired pedagogue. I was utterly enthralled. This was what I had hungered for.

There were about thirty students in our class. All, except me, were public school teachers who were taking the course for mandatory extra credits. Some of the participants were special education teachers working with mildly retarded school age children. Others were regular public school teachers who were hoping to earn a few easy credits in pleasant surroundings.

None, I soon learned, were interested in young children with disabilities, and none were enrolled in graduate school. It also turned out that the majority of the participants came from the local school district, and lived within reasonable driving distance, so practically no one elected to stay at the dormitory during the week. The few that did, seemed more intent on having a good time than studying. As soon as classes were ended for the day, off they went for drinks at the nearest pub. This didn't bother me one bit. On the contrary, I was pleased to have the time to read and study without interruptions.

Generally there were morning as well as afternoon classes. On the first day, however, instead of reconvening after lunch, we were divided into small groups and taken on a tour of the school. The first building that we entered had the same long, gloomy corridor that I encountered in the dormitory. At the end of the hall our guide opened a door.

"This is the day room," she said.

It was a barn: a vast, empty, rectangular room with dark wooden floors and equally dark wainscoting. Except for a pair of wooden benches, running the full length of the room on two sides, there was no furniture. A series of narrow, mesh-covered windows, placed just below the ceiling, along one wall, failed to relieve the gloom. A lone adolescent girl sat on one of the benches, her head turned towards a small black and white television that hung on the wall, above the door. It was obviously an old, malfunctioning set. The picture was barely visible through the flickering and snow on the screen.

I glanced at our guide. "It's so empty."

She shrugged. "Has to be. They're very destructive, you know."

"But what can they do here?"

"They sit, watch TV," a faint, apologetic smile, another shrug. "It's not as bad as it looks. We'll see the younger children now."

The guide pointed to a fenced area to one side of a low wooden building.

"That's the play area."

I approached the stone wall, expecting to see toys and swings, but all I saw was a large, barren, dusty yard, a compound teeming with little children. They clustered together, sitting on the ground, digging in the dirt with their fingers, picking up pebbles and pieces of debris. Some were tugging at the few remaining tufts of coarse grass. Little animals in a cage, I thought. A child looked up and saw me. I smiled. They surged forward, pushing and shoving, crowding around the fence, grasping my fingers, pulling on my sleeves. Again I was reminded of baby goats or fawns seeking handouts from visitors in a zoo. I had nothing, absolutely nothing to give them. I patted grubby cheeks, smoothed a few matted curls, and it was time to move on. I followed our leader in silence, blinking away tears.

Another building, another day room. This time it was a room in the men's residence. The same wooden benches lined the walls. The same, unreachable, mesh protected windows cast a feeble light into the area. The floor, however, was concrete, sloping slightly to a drain in the center of the room. The benches were unoccupied, but the floor space was crowded with men. A forest of men, some young and straight, some bent and gray-haired. Men who stood motionless, like trees, or swayed, also like trees, in trance-like rhythms. They wore slippers on bare feet and pajama-like garments, reminiscent of Nazi death camps. Some of the men had wet themselves, stains darkening the front of their pants. That was the reason for the concrete floor and the drain, I realized. We didn't enter the room. We took turns peeking through an opened doorway, then turned away. *What next?* I wondered with a tremor of dread.

Next came the women's hall and yet another day room. Once again I saw the bare floor, the covered windows, the wooden benches. Unlike the men, the women overflowed the benches, crowding together like starlings on a cold day. The center of the room was empty. We entered and trooped across to a door on the other side. Locked within themselves, the women took no notice of us. I walked slowly, trailing behind my companions. Then I saw her. A young woman, with short brown hair and a pretty face. She had jammed herself into a corner, where the bench abutted a back wall. She sat, impassive as a statue, legs drawn up, arms encircling her knees, and she was naked, completely nude, except for a tiny, lavender, flower-sprigged Peter-Pan collar that girded her slender neck like a necklace. On the bench and on the floor beneath her feet were mouse-nests of minutely shredded fabric, all that remained of her clothing. Seeing all of this, I visualized this young woman, sitting in her corner, as the hours passed, meticulously and tirelessly ripping her dress to pieces, and I was infinitely moved by her beauty and naked vulnerability.

I had witnessed such shredding of one's garments before. Once while I was still supervising the preschool for children with disabilities, I visited a woman who had an emotionally disturbed daughter, whom I had not met before. The girl was nine or ten years old. Except for a certain shyness in her manner, she appeared normal. I noticed that she was wearing an apron over her jeans and sweater. As Mrs. Leong and I sat down to talk, Lisa took a chair across the room and began fiddling with the hem of her apron. When I glanced at the child again, a few minutes later, she was ripping a corner of her garment into infinitesimal shreds. By the time we finished our conversation, the apron had been completely destroyed.

"This is why I let her wear aprons," Mrs. Leong explained in answer to my unspoken question. "If I didn't she would be tearing up her clothes, and that's harder to replace."

We were led to yet another building. A hospital, our guide informed us. We marched up a flight of stairs and entered a bright medium-sized room. I saw white walls, six white hospital cribs, white sheets, white bed covers and on each white pillow an enormous head. Human heads, each head as large as a beer keg. I stifled a scream, the wild urge to flee in terror from this science fiction nightmare. The heads were egg-shaped, immense domes, two, three, four times larger than a normal head. Like an egg these gigantic craniums tapered downward and revealed, tiny wizened faces. Beneath the faces lay the stunted, emaciated bodies of bedridden children, with necks as fragile as the naked throats of newly-hatched nestlings.

Something touched me. A withered little hand, poking through a guard rail, brushed against my skirt. I turned and looked into a pair of gentle, sky-blue eyes. The lips moved, I heard a voice, a whisper like the rustle of fallen leaves.

"What's your name?"

I approached the bed and replied.

"What's your name?" I asked in turn.

A whispered sigh, a breeze stirring dry leaves. "Violet."

A thin, translucent finger pointed to my purse.

"What's in there?"

I showed her. I took out a comb, my wallet, pencils, lipstick. I pulled out a compact and opened it. Violet looked into the mirror and smiled.

"I hope it's sunny tomorrow," she whispered.

"Why?"

"We go for a walk when it's sunny."

"That will be nice," I agreed, wondering what the child meant.

How could Violet or any of these children maintain the monstrous burden of their heads in an upright position? How could they possibly go for a walk?"

A few days later this puzzle was solved when I encountered a parade of hospital attendants pushing high-wheeled wooden vehicles that looked like peddlers' carts. Each cart carried a blanket, a pillow and a child. As the procession passed, I caught sight of Violet. She lay on her back, her eyes partially closed, her face lifted to the sun, a rapt, half-smile on her lips. I was glad for Violet, glad that it was a sunny day and that she was going for a "walk."

While I was still talking to Violet in the ward, an aide, an attractive teenaged girl came in, carrying food on a tray. She sat down beside one of the cribs and began gently spoon feeding the grotesque head that lay there. I watched, touched by her smiling face and her loving manner.

When we left the hospital I asked our guide about Violet.

"How old is she?"

"Thirteen," came the reply. Judging by her size I thought that Violet was probably five.

Violet and the other children in the ward were victims of hydrocephalus. The term hydrocephalus generally refers to condition in which water (hydro) builds up in volume inside the head (cephalus). This abnormal accumulation of cerebrospinal fluid (not actually "water") can, without treatment, result in the grotesquely enlarged heads that I had seen. Under normal circumstances this cerebrospinal fluid serves a vital function. Acting as a liquid shock absorber it prevents all, except the most severe blows to the head, from injuring the brain. It also keeps the brain tissues moist, and flushes away waste products from tissues in and around the brain. Additionally it supplies the brain with essential proteins and chemicals, similar to those found in the blood.

The cerebrospinal fluid is produced, circulated and returned to the bloodstream through something that is called the ventricular system which consists of four ventricles. A ventricle is a term used to describe natural spaces or compartments inside the brain. Small passages connect the ventricles in the same way that tunnels might connect a series of caves. Normally a delicate balance is maintained between the production, circulation and reabsorption of the cerebrospinal fluid. With the perfect precision of a well-functioning machine this balance is maintained throughout life.

Unfortunately errors occur in nature, and occasionally a child is born with a malfunctioning ventricular system. Although there may be a number of reasons for this defect, the malfunction is a blockage somewhere within the ventricular system. This blockage impedes drainage and absorption of the fluid. Since the body does not have the ability to slow down or stop the production of cerebrospinal fluid when a blockage occurs, the fluids accumulate relentlessly, growing in volume and pressure leading to the horrendous distention of the skull and the chronic condition of hydrocephalus.

When Violet and her peers were born, there was no treatment for hydrocephalus. Like Violet, children with this condition were doomed. Today, however, hydrocephalus can be prevented by a simple and reliable shunting procedure. A thin, plastic tube about the size of an ink tube inside an ink pen, is passed from one of the ventricles, under the skin, to the abdominal cavity. There the draining excessive fluid is naturally absorbed. A tiny valve inside the shunt controls the direction of flow and maintains normal fluid pressure inside the brain.

Unwilling to make further conversation, I fell behind, walking slightly apart from my fellow classmates. It appeared that we were heading back towards the dormitory. Exhausted by the emotional strain of the afternoon, I hope this was so. Would I ever be able to come to terms with what this glimpse of the hidden world of mentally retardation had revealed to me, I wondered miserably and fervently hoped that the tour was over and that no further horrors lay in store. Then, just as I was beginning to believe that my ordeal was indeed coming to an end, our guide turned into the entrance to a small wooden building. My pulse quickened with a sense of panic.

"No more," I pleaded silently. *"Please, no more, not today."*

Blissfully unaware of my distress, our guide opened a door and called out cheerfully.

"This way, ladies. Please step inside. This is the observation room."

Tense with dread, I filed into a dimly lit area that looked like a long, narrow box with a large window on one side. Still dreading what I might discover, I obediently stepped up to the window and looked through the glass.

"This is a one way mirror," I heard our guide explain. "We can look in, but the children on the inside see only a mirror. As long as it is dark in the observation room, they can't see us. This way we can observe the classroom without distracting the pupils."

I was so intent on trying to assimilate what I saw, that for a moment her words didn't register. Then the key words, "classroom" and "pupils" reached my consciousness, and a shiver of recognition like a current of electricity, streaked through my body. This very morning, our instructor, Dr. Etzel, told us about an experimental educational program at Rainier. Developmentally delayed children in the program were learning to read, write and do arithmetic.

"How is that possible?" I questioned her. "People who are mentally retarded can't do those things."

Dr. Etzel smiled. "Apparently they can. Just because traditional methods of instruction have failed, doesn't necessarily mean that mentally deficient children are incapable of learning. The potential may be there, our task is to unlock that potential."

"But how?" I questioned again, "How can this be done?"

"Dr. Sidney W. Bijou* from the psychology department at the University of Washington is responsible for the program I described. Perhaps he'll find the answer."

"That would be a miracle!" I exclaimed.

"Yes, it would," Dr. Etzel agreed.

And now, as I stood in the dimly lit observation room, I remembered Dr. Etzel's words. Were we indeed about to witness a miracle: retarded children in an academic setting? I moved close to the window.

What I saw was indeed a classroom, ten or twelve school-age children sitting at individual desks. Some, I could see were working on arithmetic problems, adding, subtracting, dividing. Others were matching words to pictures, and yet another group was printing the names of pictured objects. Two teachers moved up and down the rows of pupils, checking their work, offering praise, encouragement, rewarding correct responses with a smile, a pat, or with tokens that were dropped into plastic cups that had been placed on the desks. At the end of the class period the children exchanged tokens for a small prize: a pencil, a toy, a comic book or candy, depending upon the number of tokens that had been earned. Charts on the wall graphically displayed individual pupil progress.

These teaching techniques were based upon principles of learning and behavior as outlined by B. F. Skinner*. Dr. Bijou and his colleagues were among the first to apply these principles to the education of the mentally retarded. The beauty of this approach is that it virtually guarantees success. Each new task that the pupil is required to learn is based upon a prerequisite skill that has already been mastered. Learning becomes the mastery of a series of steps, a process not unlike that of mounting a staircase that leads to an ultimate objective. Feedback in the form of praise or tangible reinforcement (tokens), as each small step is achieved provides feedback, motivation and encouragement and a sense of accomplishment which retarded children generally lack.

Through such programs and research Dr. Bijou and his colleagues were proving that even the most severely limited individuals are capable of learning. Learning, by definition, is the ability to exhibit a skill that was not in a person's repertoire of behavior prior to specific instruction. The first time an infant repeats the word, mama, learning has taken place. The first time a severely retarded child, whom you have been teaching how to feed himself, succeeds in grasping a spoon independently, something that he or she never managed to do before, learning has occurred, even though the final goal of self-feeding may require many more instructional sessions to achieve. Too many public school special education programs fail to take into account these basic principles: instruction for children with learning differences must rely upon the hierarchy of many discrete steps. Thus, grasping a spoon, is but the first step in many leading to the final goal of self-feeding. The steps that lie between the first and the last would include dipping the spoon into the food, picking the food up on the spoon, raising the spoon to the mouth, and so on. Too often, teachers worry more about a child's cognitive processes than about their own instructional techniques.

"How can I teach a retarded child," teachers asked, "if I can't tell what he's thinking?"

"How can I teach a child, if he can't answer my questions?"

"How is it possible to teach anyone who doesn't "want" to learn?"

The behavioral approach to education, espoused by Dr. Bijou and others, including myself, circumvent these problems by being concerned only with a pupil's observable responses. In other words, if a child places the word apple on a picture of that fruit, selecting the correct word from several other words, the teacher can conclude that the desired discrimination and association have been achieved, learning has occurred, and one need not concern oneself with the student's mental process nor with the fact that the child may be nonverbal and unable to say "apple."

Too often adults expect a child to perform tasks that have little appeal, reasoning that the sole satisfaction of doing what is expected of him should provide sufficient motivation. Although many normal children do indeed acquire this inner motivation early in life, the high rate of high school drop outs and failing students suggests that even normal children may have difficulty becoming intrinsically self-motivated. This feeling of inner satisfaction that comes from a job well done, is even more difficult to develop in the pupils with special needs. Many developmentally delayed children are physically weak, their energy levels too low to generate any degree of enthusiasm for work or activities that make demands on their physical and mental capabilities. Even more significant is the fact that children with disabilities have experienced far more failures than successes in their lives. The very fact of their birth, is in fact, a failure. The failure to be born normal and healthy, the failure to fulfill the expectations of expectant parents, puts such a child at a disadvantage from the very beginning. A failure from the start, the atypical infant, without proper early intervention, continues to fail as he passes the anticipated milestones of sitting, standing, walking, talking without achieving them.

The goal of behaviorally based, special education programs, such as the one conceived by Dr. Bijou, is to create learning environments in which developmentally delayed pupils can experience success. Therefore, as I observed, until patterns of self-motivation and inner satisfaction are established, each correct response, each new achievement, however small, is acknowledged and rewarded with praise and concrete symbols of success such as tokens and treats.

Some people argue that such rewards amount to bribery[6] and don't belong in a classroom. I will not repeat the argument of why this method can be an indispensable teaching tool. Perhaps it is sufficient to point out that although we may, as adults, be motivated to work hard at our jobs for the sole satisfaction of achievement, who can deny that a merit raise or a bonus greatly enhances our feelings of self-esteem and motivates us to further effort.

Behind the observation glass, the class period had come to an end. Beaming, clutching their earned pencils and comic books, the children trooped out of the room. Then we too were dismissed. We stepped out of the school house and stood blinking in the sunshine.

'I'll leave you now," said our guide.

"Thanks for the tour," we chorused.

She gave a wave with her hand and disappeared around a corner. It was time to disperse.

"Anyone going back to the dorm?" I asked my companions. No one else was heading in that direction.

"See you tomorrow, then."

"Tomorrow," they echoed, heading for the parking lot.

I retraced my steps, thinking about all that I had seen and experienced this day. My early morning departure from home seemed to have happened eons ago. Severed from all that had been familiar, thoughts, ideas, beliefs, I felt adrift upon a chartless sea. *Would I ever find firm footing again? And if I did would I be the same person I was ten hours ago?* As I passed the imposing facade of a residence hall I remembered the desolation within, and then I remembered the classroom and the promise it held.

Was that indeed a promise for a brighter future? Would the day come, I wondered, when all children, the normal as well as the retarded, would have equal rights to an education? Would educational programs, such as I had seen, become the magic key to hidden potentials? If this were true, would the day come when gloomy ward rooms, crowded with vegetating men and vacant-eyed women, would stand empty, no longer holding pens for discarded humanity? Would little children no longer be condemned to grub in the dirt, herded together like lost lambs in a barren corral? What about children like Violet, who would come to their aid? Would the medical community find a cure? Was there hope? Would I live to see this vision become a reality?

I pondered these questions, not yet fully realizing that what I had witnessed in the classroom was indeed the beginning, the first stirrings of a revolution, the emergence of a new era in the lives of the physically and mentally disabled people. Nor did I know that I too would play a role in making this dream a reality.

Chapter Five
Manipulative Moppets

PRINCESS LUCY

Like a family of sleek, well-fed penguins, the Leonards, father, mother, two teenaged sons, and stocky three-year-old Lucy, filed into the building. Of medium height, with thick, neatly groomed glossy black hair, rounded torsos and slightly protruding abdomens, they looked like pleasant, complacent, self-satisfied people. As I came forward to greet them, Lucy broke rank and toddled across the lobby to a classroom door.

Pointing an imperious finger at the door she said "Ung."

Mr. Leonard pushed past me and hurriedly opened the door. Lucy marched in with the aplomb of royalty. Her father gave a little shrug and smiled apologetically.

"She doesn't like to wait," he explained.

I smiled in return and led them into the classroom. We seated ourselves at a low preschool table and began going over Lucy's records. Left to herself, Lucy roamed about the room, exploring her new surroundings. Every few minutes she pointed to something that was out of reach and said "Ung." As if stung a family member sprung up to hand her the desired toy.

The conference dragged on. Lucy's brothers were becoming bored. Noting their discomfort I suggested that they wait in the playground. Obviously pleased, the boys went outside. Lucy continued her wanderings about the room. Finally she approached her mother's chair.

"Ung," said Lucy.

Engrossed in our conversation, Mrs. Leonard didn't respond immediately.

"Ung!" repeated Lucy in a louder tone.

"What is it, darling?" asked Mama.

"Ung, ung!" persisted Lucy with increasing impatience.

Mr. Leonard looked concerned.

"Come on, honey, show Daddy what you want."

"UNG!" screeched Lucy. Her face turned red. She stamped her foot.

"UNG! UNG!" The piercing cries sounded like a siren.

"Maybe she's hungry," guessed her mother, fumbling in her purse, and bringing out a plastic-wrapped treat.

"Cookie, you want a cookie?"

"Ung!" screamed the child and batted the offering away.

The shrill cries resumed.

"I think she wants to go outside," said Father. He rose to his feet.

"Come, baby, Daddy will take you outside."

The shrieks stopped. Taking her father's hand, Lucy trotted beside him, a sweet, docile little girl, but I could hardly keep from laughing at the smug expression on her perky, round face.

"Does Lucy say anything besides "ung?" I asked.

Mrs. Leonard shook her head. "Not yet, but we're pretty good at figuring out what she wants. Although we do have to be on our toes. Lucy gets pretty upset if we don't guess what she wants right away."

I restrained a smile. "Yes, I could see that ... have you tried teaching her to speak. A few words, perhaps?"

Mrs. Leonard sighed. "Yes, I tried, in the beginning. We all tried, but it's no use. I know she could speak if she wanted to, but obviously she doesn't. Lucy has a mind of her own. You just can't make her do what she doesn't want to do."

"We'll see about that," I thought to myself.

"It may be different in a school situation," I said out loud. "Beside," I smiled, to take the sting out of my words. "You're so clever at figuring out what she wants, Lucy has no real need to say anything, does she?"

"But — but how would you make her talk?" Mrs. Leonard looked frightened, her voice dropped to a whisper. "You ... you're not going to *punish* her?"

"Most certainly not! We don't punish children. It is simply a matter of structuring the environment in such a way that learning occurs."

Mrs. Leonard looked at me blankly.

"You'll see how it works, once Lucy gets into the program."

At this point Lucy ran into the room, followed by Mr. Leonard and the boys. She was clutching something to her chest that her father seemed intent on taking away from her.

"Lucy, baby, come on, honey, give them back to Daddy," he pleaded.

Lucy was backing away from him, shaking her head.

"Sweetheart," he begged, "give them to me. I can't drive the car without them."

Mrs. Leonard chimed in. "Give Daddy the car keys, darling. We can all go home and have a nice big lunch."

Lucy gave a huge, mischievous grin, laughed and darted around a corner to an adjoining room. Picking up a small picture book, I followed after Lucy and her parents.

Lucy was behind a door, backed up against the wall. She was no longer giggling. Her face was set. Another tantrum was brewing. Father and mother stood looking at her helplessly. It was a stand off.

"Excuse me." Impatient with such shenanigans, I brushed past the Leonards.

"Daddy needs the keys,' I said firmly. In one quick motion I plucked the keys from her hands and gave her the book. "Here's a book for you, Lucy. You can look at it on the way home."

Lucy opened her mouth to shriek, then closed it. The book caught her attention. I took her hand.

"Show me Daddy's car."

The child obeyed, leading me to the front entrance.

The Leonards followed, grinning sheepishly.

"How did you do it?" Mr. Leonard asked.

"I was sure she'd scream," added his wife.

I laughed. "I think I took her by surprise. Anyway I'm glad it worked. It may not next time. Then I'll have to try something else."

Nevertheless I was pleased that I had won my first skirmish with Lucy, never dreaming to what extent she would challenge my patience and ingenuity in the days ahead.

The morning I met Lucy was the first day of Fall quarter at the University of Washington. Summer classes at Rainier State school ended a few weeks ago, and I was now on campus, ready to begin my second quarter of studies and my new job.

The room which Lucy explored was one of two preschool classrooms situated in a campus building called the Developmental Psychology Laboratory, DPL, for short. Staffed by skilled teachers and serving normal three and four year old youngsters, the purpose of the DPL preschools was to give the children a quality experience and at the same time to offer psychology majors the opportunity of studying typical child behavior. Psychology students, coming into the classroom, sat unobtrusively around the edges of the room to record their observations. All aspects of child behavior and development: play skills, aggressive behaviors, language and cognitive development were analyzed. Direct interaction with the children was forbidden, as a result the preschoolers quickly learned to ignore the students.

Dr. Bijou, whose program I had observed at Rainier, also happened to be director of the Developmental Psychology Laboratory. Mrs. Florence Harris*, a woman in her sixties, an outstanding instructor and pedagogue, who strongly resembled Eleanor Roosevelt in manner and appearance, directed the preschool programs. This particular school year, in addition to the classes for normal children, Dr. Bijou and Mrs. Harris initiated a new, highly structured, intensive remedial program, especially designed to serve three preschoolers with severe language and development deficits. Three teachers, of which I was one, were hired to work with these youngsters on a one-to-one basis.

Although Dr. Etzel was our main instructor at the Rainier School workshop, Bijou and Harris were frequent guest speakers. As a result I had the opportunity of meeting them on several occasions. Apparently they were pleased with my work, because before the summer classes ended, I was offered a teaching position in the newly established remedial classroom. It was a part-time morning job which left my afternoons free for class attendance and studying. Naturally, I was delighted with the offer, not so much for the salary that I would receive, although by 1965 standards it was very adequate, as for the welcome opportunity of working directly under Florence Harris and Sidney Bijou whom I had come to admire very much.

After meeting Lucy, I was thrilled when she was assigned to me. The little girl intrigued me, and I looked forward to working with her. Confident in my ability to help her acquire speech, I gave no thought to the possibility of unforeseen difficulties.

The remedial program began smoothly. In three weeks we were scheduled to begin individual speech training sessions with our pupils, meanwhile our task was to establish rapport between teacher and child, and to concentrate on developing desirable classroom behaviors. Lucy and I became friends and she readily adjusted to the preschool routine. Although Lucy still pointed and grunted to make her wants known, there had been no tantrums. Apparently the school activities kept her so happily occupied that it was no longer necessary for her to demand constant attention.

On the first day of school, however, something happened that made me realize there was one thing I had to teach Lucy immediately, without delay. The morning began with outdoor games in the large, fenced area adjoining the building. To reach the play court the children left the classroom by the back door, crossed a small porch and descended four steps. My fellow teachers and the two boys, under their supervision, led the way. Lucy, who was the youngest, lagged behind. After helping her with her jacket and zipper, I opened the door. Head high, a royal princess on parade, Lucy marched to the edge of the porch, and then, to my utter horror, stepped off into space. I flung myself forward and somehow managed to grab her solid little body an instant before she slammed, head first, onto a concrete sidewalk.

I sank down on the bottom step, clutching Lucy, my heart pounding, weak with relief. Blissfully unaware of the averted disaster, Lucy gave a bright smile, revealing an even row of tiny baby teeth, and toddled off towards a swing. A few minutes later, regaining my composure, I brought Lucy back to the steps in order to assess her step-climbing ability. I soon discovered that unless I held her hand, Lucy could neither ascend nor descend the stairs independently, she didn't even know enough to hang on to the handrail. This should not have surprised me. Her records showed that Lucy was indeed delayed in many areas of her development. Although the cause was unknown, psychological tests confirmed that in some respects Lucy functioned at a seventeen month level. A typical toddler doesn't walk up and down steps at that age, so Lucy's inability to manage steps was to be expected.

Normally toddlers learn to ascend a stairway by crawling on their hands and knees. Descending, if they are allowed to do so independently, some children learn to bump downward from step to step on their bottoms. These were the strategies my own children used in mastering the feat of going up and down stairs, and this is what I decided to teach Lucy to do.

Enticed by a toy that I placed out of reach on the porch, Lucy quickly learned to drop to her knees and to crawl up the stairs. Next, reversing the process, I taught Lucy to sit down on the edge of the porch and then to bump down the steps as I had seen my own toddlers do. To my delight Lucy readily perfected both maneuvers and within a few days she was so skilled at ascending and descending independently that it was safe for her to go up and down without close supervision. Later I would show her how to walk the steps properly, but for the time being I was satisfied.

Three weeks passed and at last it was time to begin speech lessons with our pupils. Each teacher and her assigned child were scheduled to spend fifteen to twenty minutes a day in a one-to-one session in a small therapy room, equipped with a one-way mirror. In the beginning, since I was a novice, Florence Harris, and sometimes, Dr. Bijou, monitored my work with Lucy, observing us through the one-way glass and directing their instructions to me through a microphone in my ear.

The training program, as these lessons were called, was based upon a set of uniform, predetermined procedures. We, the teachers, were not speech therapists. Research[7] had shown, however, that a systematic application of these procedures, was an effective first step towards language acquisition among nonverbal children.

Sitting in a chair, and facing a teacher across a small table, each child was expected to progress through the following series of steps. Specifically, each child would, on command:

1. Sit quietly;
2. Look at the teacher;
3. Manipulate toys;
4. Respond to commands of look, take, put and give;
5. Imitate gestures;
6. Imitate sounds;
7. Imitate speech sounds;

8. Imitate the naming of objects and pictures;

9. Name objects and pictures spontaneously;

10. Initiate speech sounds and words;

11. Initiate speech sounds and words outside the therapy room; in the classroom, at home, etc.

The behavior of the teacher also followed a predetermined set of procedures. Briefly, depending upon the child's responses, the teacher does the following:

1. Gives the predetermined command;

2. Praises and rewards each correct response if it occurs within fifteen seconds;

3. If the desired response doesn't occur, repeats the command, helps the child to respond correctly, and praises the effort. For example if a child doesn't pick up a toy on the command "take," the teacher repeats the command and at the same time places the child's hand over the toy;
4. If the child tantrums or becomes uncooperative the teacher drops her head and ignores the child for thirty seconds. If the tantrum continues, the teacher exits from the therapy room, leaving the child alone until the crying stops. The instant the child becomes quiet, the teacher returns, praises the child for quiet behavior, and resumes the training session.

Lucy and I sailed through the first four steps of the program without a hitch. She sat quietly in a high chair — a regular preschool chair proved too low. She made eye-contact when I said "look." She smiled when

I praised her and eagerly dropped poker chips into an empty mayonnaise jar. When I brought out the toys, small rubber animals, blocks and cars, she responded to commands of "take," "put," or "give."

Thus the first week of training ended on a positive note. I was full of praise for Lucy and Harris and Bijou praised me. The following Monday I would begin step five: imitation of gestures. Imitation, the ability to observe and to reproduce actions as performed by someone else, is an extremely important aspect of learning. Since children with delays tend to be much slower than their normal peers in acquiring this essential developmental skill, I was especially eager to begin this new phase of the training program with Lucy.

The reason the ability to imitate plays such an important role in learning, is that imitation fosters awareness. In order to imitate, a child must focus on what is going on. The ability to imitate requires attention and awareness, key elements in learning.

It would be impossible to list all the general and specific kinds of learning that occur through the imitation of modeled behaviors. This, in fact, is a type of learning that continues throughout life. Even as adults we continue to learn new behaviors by observing and imitating the actions of others.

Children, like adults, learn many self-help, social, academic and play skills through imitation. In all of these areas the ability to imitate is helpful, but not crucial. For language development, however, the ability to imitate is absolutely essential. A child who hears, but is unable to reproduce (imitate) the sounds of the words that he hears, will never be able to talk. All children in the world learn to walk, eat and play in basically similar ways, only the spoken languages are different. A child or anyone, for that matter, learns to speak only the language that he hears: the sound which he can imitate.

Lucy did not speak. I had yet to hear her make a vocal sound other than the threatening "ung" which was more of a grunt than a vocalization. Yet I knew that she was not deaf, and from her responses to my simple commands I knew that she had some understanding of the meaning of words. Somehow I would have to bridge the gap between what Lucy could hear and understand, her receptive language, and the ability to say the words that she heard in order to communicate. This was the ultimate goal of the training program and my task. This was why I had to teach her to imitate.

Monday came. Anxious to resume our training sessions, I led Lucy to the therapy room and seated her in the high chair. After a brief review of the preceding week's exercises, I planned to model a few simple motor actions such as tapping the table top and clapping hands, that Lucy could imitate.

Repeating what had been so successful the previous week, I leaned forward and gave a command. "Look at me."

Instead of complying good-naturedly, Lucy folded her arms across her chest and glared.

"Go-od ... girl," I said hesitantly, not sure whether or not I should praise such a belligerent stare. Nevertheless, eye-contact had been made. I handed her a chip. Lucy ignored me. I dropped the chip into the jar.

"Look at me." I tried again.

Arms crossed, Lucy turned aside. After waiting the required fifteen seconds, I placed my hands on her face to direct it towards me, and repeated the command.

Lucy jerked away. "UNG!"

The mike buzzed in my ear. "Time out!" hissed Mrs. Harris.

I dropped my head and ignored Lucy for thirty seconds.

"Okay," said Harris.

I selected a toy, Lucy's favorite, a rubber horse, and placed it on the table top.

"Take the horse, Lucy."

She sat, grim as a carving on a totem pole.

Again I waited fifteen seconds, and then, repeating the cue, reached for Lucy's hand in order to guide her through the desired response. As I touched her arm, Lucy snatched the toy out of my fingers and threw it forcefully across the room.

"UNG!" she screamed at the top of her voice, kicking her feet and striking a sharp blow to my left knee.

"Leave!" Harris shouted in my ear.

Rubbing my knee, I grabbed my notebook and hobbled out of the room. Bijou and Harris were in the observation booth.

Imprisoned in her chair Lucy kicked and screamed. Her face was scarlet, shuddering gasps punctuated her shrieks. I could hardly stand it. I had become very fond of Lucy.

"Oh, that poor child! We can't let this go on. She'll make herself sick! Please, Mrs. Harris, let me go in. She's just a baby," I pleaded.

Harris laid a restraining hand on my arm. "You must wait until she's quiet. That child has been manipulating her parents and brothers all her life. If you give in now she'll know that she can manipulate you, too."

Dr. Bijou's warm, olive black eyes, looked at me with sympathy.

"Don't you want to help that child?"

"Oh, yes, I do. But not like this ... What if she's in pain or frightened? How can I leave her like this?" I was ready to cry myself.

"I assure you she's all right."

I glanced at the clock in the therapy room. Only two minutes had passed since I walked out. I thought

Lucy had been crying for hours. Then as the yowling continued to reverberate through the wooden building, I heard the clatter of someone running down the stairs from the second floor. The next instant the door opened, and Dr. Rob Hawkins*, a young psychologist on Dr. Bijou's staff, entered. He carried a tape recorder and a microphone. His eyes sparkled with excitement.

"What's going on? This is the best tantrum I've ever heard. I must get it on tape! Where can I plug in my machine? Is there an outlet in this room?"

"No," I replied, "not in here. There's one in the therapy room, in back of the high chair."

"I guess I'll just have to sneak in."

"No, don't!" cautioned Florence Harris.

"It will be all right." Intent upon his objective Rob dropped to his knees, and, after opening the door a crack, began creeping towards the electrical outlet.

"WA—!" As if someone had flicked off a switch, Lucy's howl died in mid-air. She had spotted Rob's maneuvers. With the cold disdain of a queen observing the awkward progress of a crawling insect, Lucy regarded the man on the floor. I, in turn, studied Lucy. Her cheeks were pink, but there were no tears, even her breathing appeared to be no more agitated than if she had been sitting quietly, playing, with her toys.

"You were right!" I turned to Mrs. Harris, "It was just an act!"

"I told you."

"What a clever child." I couldn't help admiring Lucy.

"Shoot!" said Rob, chagrined. "I blew it. I did so want to get a really great tantrum on tape."

Bijou patted him on the shoulder. "There will be other opportunities, I'm sure. But next time, don't go barging into a therapy room when a child is in 'timeout.'

"Yes, I'm sorry. I hope I didn't damage the procedures."

Secretly glad that the distraction had put an end to the tantrum, I gave him a smile, and returned to the therapy room. I closed the door, sat down and gave my command.

"Look at me, Lucy."

She met my eyes and smiled expectantly.

"Good, girl!" I handed her a chip. She dropped it into the jar.

I tapped the table with my hand. "Do this."

Lucy looked at me then gave a tentative little tap.

"Oh, good, girl!" I cried delightedly and another chip dropped into the container.

"Once more!" I tapped the table. Lucy tapped in return.

"Oh, Lucy, good for you. You tapped the table!"

Lucy grinned, pleased with herself. Equally pleased, I ended the session and lifted Lucy down from her chair.

The training program continued. Occasionally Lucy balked and refused to respond, but the incidents were easily resolved with a time-out procedure during which I dropped my head and refused to interact with her for thirty seconds. There were no more screaming tantrums like the one that sent me from the room. Yet, despite Lucy's general cooperativeness, progress was slow. Lucy learned to tap the table but it was another week before she learned to imitate hand-clapping, and two more before she imitated touching her head or her nose, her lips, her chin. Starting out with the large movements of tapping and clapping I was gradually focusing Lucy's attention to the movement of her lips and jaw as one of prerequisite steps to sound production.

At last when classes resumed after Christmas break, I was ready to begin vocal imitations. My initial goal was to teach Lucy to repeat basic vowel sounds. We began with the "ah" sound.

I placed a finger on my chin, dropped my jaw and said "ah."

Dutifully Lucy placed a finger on her chin, and opened her mouth. There was no sound.

After praising Lucy for trying, we repeated the exercise. Still no sound, not even a gurgle. I presented the activity three more times, and as before Lucy imitated my gesture, but made no attempt at vocalization. Not wishing to make the mistake of boring Lucy with numerous repetitions I moved on to a series of other exercises, pairing a number of actions with other vowel sounds.

"Eye," I said, using the word for the vowel sound of "i", and pointing to my eye.

Lucy repeated the gesture, but made no sound. I picked up a doll that I had brought with me, and pointed to the doll's eye.

Lucy smiled and pointed, but that was all. I made a circle with my fingers and said O. And yet again Lucy was silent.

This went on for several days. I was beginning to despair. It seemed that I would never succeed in eliciting a vocal sound from Lucy. Then one day, as Lucy again touched her chin, opened her mouth, I reached across the table and gave her a slight poke to the diaphragm.

"A-ack," croaked Lucy in spite of herself.

"Lucy!" I hugged her.

And once more, as Lucy imitated me, placing a finger on her chin, opening her mouth, I gave a little poke.

Lucy grunted, "ah."

We did it again and again, finger on chin, mouth open, poke.

Each time Lucy made an "ah" sound.

Finally, for the last time, I touched my chin, dropped the jaw, said "ah," but as Lucy repeated my gestures, I withheld the poke.

"Ah," said Lucy loud and clear.

I could have wept with joy. Lucy had consciously made her first vocal imitation. She had learned a new skill!

Some time later Mrs. Leonard reported to me that Lucy had begun "reading" the *Readers' Digest.* Poking her finger at the words on the page, Lucy repeatedly said "ah, ah, ah."

Slowly one letter at a time, Lucy mastered the vowel sounds. And each time before she uttered the desired sound I had to invent a new gimmick. Once in desperation, as she struggled over the "oo" sound, I snatched off my shoe and waved it over my head.

"Sh-oo," I exclaimed.

Lucy raised her foot, reached over the high chair tray and pulled off her sneaker.

"Oo!" she said.

Another time I brought a toy telephone to our room, holding the receiver to my ear, I called out "Hi!"

After a few trials Lucy, too, learned to say "Hi" into the phone.

We moved on to consonants. By holding her nose Lucy learned to say "n". Clamping her lips together, Lucy finally came out with an "m". But before she could do that, I again had to give a poke to her diaphragm to force the correct sound through her closed lips.

After Lucy had learned to say a few of the basic consonants I began teaching her how to blend letters together, another step towards the utterance of words.

The first word on my list was mama. Normal babies say "ma-ma" early in their development, so I decided this was an appropriate choice.

I clamped my lips.

Lucy did likewise.

I said "m".

Lucy complied.

Finger on chin, mouth open, I said "ah."

So did Lucy.

I said "ma," making the usual movements with my hand and lips.

Lucy imitated my gestures and said "m-ah."

It took almost four weeks before Lucy learned to blend the two sounds together, and finally say "ma-ma" without the gestures.

Nevertheless we were making progress. Now that we had overcome the hurdle of blending consonants and vowels with mama, subsequent words such as baby, apple, bye-bye were learned and spoken much more readily.

By the end of Spring quarter, and the end of the program, Lucy had a vocabulary of forty words. She could name pictures in a book, animals and objects in her environment. She could ask for juice, milk, cookies.

Moreover Lucy was talking to herself in a constant stream of babbling. Like an infant who spends hours gooing and gurgling, Lucy was experimenting with vocalizations. She had discovered the joy and power of communication. When a word failed her, she vocalized, making up her own words.

Lucy did not return to the DPL preschool in the fall. Much to my regret, Dr. Bijou left the University of Washington to teach at another institution. A new director, with other interests came to take his place. The remedial program was not resumed. I was rehired as a head teacher in the laboratory preschool class for normal three year olds.

Before Lucy left DPL, I met with her parents, outlined the training program, supplied them with pictures and books and urged them to continue her program at home. Later that summer, anxious about Lucy's progress I visited the Leonards at their house. Lucy was still manipulating the household. Again "Ung" was a much repeated sound. I was saddened by what I saw, but I had to accept the fact that the Leonards were a very loving, but easy going family. It was easier for them to comply to Lucy's infantile demands, than to expend the kind of energy it took to teach Lucy the words that she could now speak, and to modify her undesirable behaviors. Old habits, I realized, are hard to break, for adults as it is for children. Still I did hear Lucy use some of the words that I had taught her, and she was still babbling. That gave me some hope for her future. I encouraged the Leonards to enroll Lucy in nursery school. I hope they followed my advice.

TIMID TREVOR

"I can't even go to the bathroom!" The voice on the telephone was that of a young, agitated woman.

"Is it a medical problem?" I asked.

'No, it's not a medical problem!"

"Then what ... ?"

"I can't leave him for a second."

"Who?"

"Trevor."

"Trevor?" I echoed foolishly, groping for enlightenment.

"My little boy."

"Why can't ...

"Because, he'll fall and hurt his head!"

I thought I was beginning to understand. "Trevor has seizures?"

"Oh, no!"

"Can you ... ah ... be a little more specific?"

"He turns blue and falls to the floor."

"Have you taken him to a doctor?"

"Many times, to several doctors. They all say there's nothing wrong. They say Trevor is stubborn. They tell me to ignore him. How can I, when he turns blue and falls to the floor!"

"How old is Trevor?" I asked, still trying to figure out what it was that we were supposed to be discussing.

"Two and a half."

Aha. Finally the conversation was beginning to make some sense.

"Young children do that sometimes," I counseled soothingly, "they get mad and hold their breath, but I've never heard of a child actually fainting. Usually children begin breathing in spite of themselves. It's virtually impossible to hold one's breath to the point of blacking out."

"Trevor can. That's where you and the doctors are wrong."

"Are you sure, about the fainting, I mean?"

"After what happened? Are you kidding? Of course, I'm sure."

"So, what did happen?"

"I did what the doctors told me to do. When Trevor started holding his breath, I ignored him, walked out of the room. He fell, just like I knew he would, hit his head on the coffee table. It took five stitches to close up the wound!"

"Gracious! When was that?"

"Two days ago."

"No wonder you're upset."

"I'm scared to death! I don't know what to do anymore. The doctor told me to talk to someone in the psychology department. Can you help me?"

"If it's a behavioral, and not a medical problem, perhaps I can," I answered, inviting her to come to the DPL the following afternoon.

After thanking me and promising to come, Trevor's mother gave me her name.

"My first name used to be Diane," she explained, "but I've changed it to Artemis."

"After the moon goddess?"

"Yeah, it's sort of closer to nature ... I dig nature, don't you?"

"Oh, yes, yes, indeed," I concurred enthusiastically.

I hung up the phone and looked out. The old cherry tree in the children's play court was in full bloom. Massive boughs, frothing with white blossoms tapped against my second story office window. It was May 1967. Three months prior I had received my Master's in Special Education. Euphoric with this achievement, I didn't foresee that within a few years I would again feel inwardly impelled to climb yet another rung up the academic ladder to obtain a Ph.D. in Early Childhood Education/Special Education. For the moment I was content, happy with my new position as a full-time employee at DPL. Although I was still head teacher for normal three-year olds, my afternoons were now devoted to research that focused on the application of behavioral principles towards modifying problem behaviors among young children. In 1967 behavior modification was as yet a relatively new approach to education, as a result everyone at DPL was encouraged to conduct carefully documented case studies in order to add to the growing literature on the subject. I loved this aspect of my job, as much for the challenge as for the personal satisfaction of helping troubled children and their parents. Trevor, I thought, might prove to be an interesting case.

The following afternoon Artemis arrived on time. She entered the now empty classroom carrying Trevor. Dressed in navy shorts and a red T-shirt, he was a slender, delicate-looking boy who clung to his mother like a tentacled sea creature. Thin arms entwined her neck, long, bare legs clasped her about the waist. His face was hidden against her shoulder, but I could see his scalp and a row of stitches where his dark, curly hair had been shaved off.

The young woman looked hot and tired, noticeably subdued in contrast to her earlier agitation.

"It's a long walk from the bus," she sighed, sinking down on a proffered chair and shifting Trevor to her lap. Tall and slender, with a pale, oval face, she wore the garb of a 1960's flower child: a long cotton skirt, a floppy embroidered blouse and sandals over bare feet. A beaded head-band circled her brow. Long, golden-brown hair flowed down her back like maple syrup.

I served paper cups of chilled apple juice. After a few sips both mother and child began to relax. Trevor slid off his mother's knee and stood leaning against her, studying me over the rim of his cup with a bright, solemn gaze. He appeared to be a perfectly normal little boy, although obviously extremely timid, for whenever I made the slightest movement in his direction, he immediately stiffened and buried his face against his mother's breast. Nevertheless, it was time to learn more about Trevor's problem. I laid a few toys on a table and gently took Trevor's hand, to lead him to the table.

He gave a sharp cry and jerked away.

"Artemis!" He clutched her skirt and took a deep gulp of air.

"He's holding his breath!" Artemis cried in anguish.

"Trevor, don't!" She scooped him up in her arms.

His face had reddened. His lips and eyes were tightly clamped.

"Oh, he's going to turn blue, I know it! Trevor! Trevor!" She was shaking him desperately. Stoically Trevor held his breath.

"May I?" I lifted Trevor out of his mother's arms and laid him on a rug a few feet away.

"Artemis!" He exclaimed in alarm, his breathing restored, and sitting up immediately. His eyes darted about the room seeking his mother.

"I'm here, Trevor."

He scrambled to his feet and ran happily to her side.

Convinced that Trevor would not separate easily from his mother, I directed Artemis to lead Trevor to the toys on the table. Instead of encouraging Trevor to sit independently on the chair that I had placed in front of the table, Artemis took the chair herself. Trevor climbed up on her lap and reached for a set of nesting cups. After he stacked the cups I held out some pegs and a peg board.

"Give me pegs," said Trevor, displaying good verbal skills.

I pointed to another child-sized chair. "Sit here, by yourself," I told him, "then you may play with the pegs," adding, as I turned to his mother, "please show Trevor where he should sit."

Artemis slid Trevor off her lap and stood up. Trevor clutched her skirt and shook his head.

"Do what the teacher says," Artemis prompted.

Trevor threw her a despairing look and took a deep breath.

"Oh!" Artemis glanced at me helplessly.

"Lay him on the floor, and walk away," I directed.

"Come back!" called Trevor, struggling to his feet.

"I will if you sit on that chair," Artemis told him, as I nodded my approval.

Trevor obeyed and Artemis sat down beside him. I placed the board and pegs on the table. Noting Trevor's fine motor skills and long attention span as he meticulously inserted the tiny pegs in even rows, I commented on his development. For the first time, Artemis' pale, anxious face brightened with a smile.

"Oh, you think so! I expect it's because I spend so much time with him. I have to, you saw what happens. He won't let me out of his sight. Besides there's no one else."

"No children to play with?"

She shook her head.

"What about yourself? Any friends your age?"

"I ... I haven't been in Seattle very long."

"Are you a single parent, perhaps?"

"No," she twisted the narrow band on her finger, sometimes I think I am, though. Jack's in Canada, near Prince Rupert, somewhere. That's why I moved to Seattle ... closer to the border."

I looked at her questioningly. A slight flush reddened her cheeks. "The draft you know."

I made no reply. She gave me a sudden, hard, defiant stare.

"Jack ... we ... don't believe in killing."

I nodded in sympathy, keenly aware of the war in Vietnam, of the controversy surrounding this conflict and my own feelings as the mother of two draft eligible sons. Artemis was still defiant.

"I'm not on welfare! Jack has a job. He sends me money!"

I nodded again and smiled at the young woman. It was time to return to Trevor's problem.

"When did Trevor start holding his breath?" I asked.

"Six months ago, Trevor had a bad cold and ear infection," she answered. Artemis told me she spent hours rocking and carrying Trevor because of his crying and fussing. Then on top of everything else, Jack slipped over the border. When Trevor wasn't crying from pain, he was calling for his father.

"Yack ... Yack ... " Artemis imitated the little boy.

"Trevor loves his daddy. He couldn't say Jack, so he called him Yack. Trevor calls us by our first names, you know."

"Yes, I noticed that," I agreed.

Artemis went on with her story.

"One night Trevor woke up with a high fever. He was crying and thrashing about in his crib, suddenly he gasped, started to choke, and stopped breathing. I was terrified. I snatched him up out of the crib, shook him, and he started breathing again."

A few days later, during a minor crying spell, the breath-holding happened again. Again Artemis picked him up and shook him. Increasingly Artemis became more and more fearful of anything that might make Trevor cry. By the time Trevor recovered from his illness, a pattern had been established. As Artemis' anxiety increased so did Trevor's control, until, as I witnessed, the slightest threat of a physical separation from his mother resulted in immediate breath-holding and the actual danger of a head injury.

"Why did you put Trevor on the floor?" she asked me.

"If he's already lying down, he can't fall and hurt himself, can he?" I replied.

Trevor, of course, was not consciously aware that he had this control over his mother. Like most young children, Trevor had a great dependency on his mother, especially since, in their isolation, he didn't have the opportunity of learning to relate to anyone else. Jack, the only other person to whom he was attached, had disappeared. Having no clear understanding of the future or the passage of time, the sudden disappearance of a parent can be an extremely frightening occurrence to a small child. Moreover Jack's departure came at a time when Trevor was particularly vulnerable to emotional stress. Illness inevitably increased his normal toddler dependency on his mother and augmented his underlying anxiety that she, too, might vanish.

The first breath-holding episode occurred during a moment of physical and emotional stress. Such episodes are sometimes attributed to neurophysical immaturity which children are expected to outgrow by age three. By the time I met Trevor, however, his breath-holding had become a learned behavior, a method by which he could very successfully prevent his mother's disappearance.

Considering Trevor's problem, I realized that I had a dual task. First it was necessary to create a situation under which Artemis could once again be in control. In order to achieve this, Artemis had to be free to ignore Trevor's breath-holding, without the fear of jeopardizing his safety. The act of placing Trevor on the floor gave her this freedom. Assured of her child's safety, she could walk away, and thereby reestablish her rightful control. Satisfied that this strategy was proving to be effective, I turned my attention to the second task. This entailed teaching Trevor that a brief separation from his mother would not result in a permanent loss. Trevor had to learn what all children must learn in order to achieve social maturity and independence: mother may leave, but mother will return.

After explaining my assumptions to Artemis, I took a sheet of paper and jotted down a hierarchy of training steps for Trevor. It was a simple plan. After setting a timer for fifteen seconds, Artemis would, as a precaution, place Trevor on the floor, and before he had a chance to protest or hold his breath, step behind a door. As soon as the timer went off, she would reappear, praise Trevor for waiting, and reassure him that when the timer rang, she would return. The goal was two-fold. The first was to increase the time of Artemis' absence from fifteen seconds to three minutes. The second goal was to reach a point when it would no longer be necessary to lay Trevor on the floor before leaving the room, because he would no longer hold his breath when it appeared that Artemis might leave his side.

Despite some reservations, Artemis agreed to my proposal. We showed a timer to Trevor and demonstrated how it worked. Then, before he could protest or hold his breath, Artemis laid him on the rug and stepped out of sight. The timer rang, she reappeared and Trevor greeted her with a smile. Greatly encouraged we repeated the exercise several more times with equal success.

"He's catching on," I told Artemis, but I also cautioned her not to rush things. Above all it was important to prevent the rise of anxiety in Trevor. Although it appeared that Trevor was able to tolerate a fifteen-second separation from his mother, a sharp increase in the length of her disappearance might create more anxiety than he could tolerate at present and would only serve to delay the learning process.

Before Trevor and Artemis left DPL, I gave her an outline of Trevor's training program and instructed her to phone me every day to report on his progress. I also introduced her to my assistant teacher, Daphne. A student in the Master's program, Daphne was a divorced mother with two small children. Still in her early twenties, Daphne was successfully managing her life as a mother, student and teacher. I believed that she would make a good role model for Artemis, and I was pleased when Daphne volunteered to visit Artemis two or three times a week to monitor Trevor's progress.

With Daphne's support and the daily phone calls Artemis and Trevor made rapid gains. The program was going so well that after two weeks I told Artemis that she could cut back on the phone calls and that Daphne would begin limiting her visits to once a week.

We no sooner put this new regime into effect when Artemis reported that Trevor had regressed to his previous behavior. He was crying, clinging and holding his breath.

"I can't believe this," said Daphne. "Last time I was there, Artemis left the room for three minutes. Trevor was so busy playing with his blocks, it wasn't even necessary to lay him on the floor. I guess I'll have to see for myself."

"I don't know what Artemis is talking about," Daphne reported the next day. "I didn't see anything wrong. Trevor behaved perfectly. I told Artemis that I'd come in a week, not any sooner. In fact, it's hardly necessary for me to come at all!"

"What did she say?" I asked.

"She began to cry. She told me how worried she was about Trevor and that she couldn't manage without my help. I don't know what's going on."

"I think I do," I answered slowly. "Artemis is manipulating *us*. She's lonely. She's trying to hold on to your companionship. As long as there's a problem with Trevor she can count on your visits ... so, she creates problems where none exist."

"We can't just drop her!"

"No," I agreed, "but we can change the contingency. We'll up the ante. We'll set new goals for Trevor. Let's get him ready for nursery school. Meanwhile you'll visit only when there's some new progress to report."

Daphne told Artemis that she would visit again as soon as Trevor was able to play by himself for four minutes. She also encouraged Artemis to seek out a local cooperative preschool where both she and Trevor would find companionship. As Artemis began concentrating on the positive aspects of Trevor's behavior, her self-confidence increased, and she became less and less dependent on Daphne's support. Eventually she stopped phoning me and Daphne's visits were discontinued.

Manipulative behavior in children as well as in adults is a means to an end. Aside from the basic need for air to breathe and food and warmth to survive, a child's other basic need is the need for attention and, as a result, control. Most manipulative behaviors are aimed at getting this attention. Children who provoke parental concern and nagging by refusing to eat, or to talk, or who cling to their mothers to the extent that Trevor did, are getting the attention they crave. When adults disregard positive behaviors, a child will find other ways of being noticed, usually through misbehavior or actions which can't be ignored. Fundamentally manipulative behaviors are harmful because they can interfere with a child's expected intellectual and social development. Manipulative behavior can also be a trap into which unsuspecting parents stumble unwittingly. Therefore it is essential for parents to recognize and to circumvent such behaviors when they occur. Once successful a child's manipulative behavior is likely to be repeated, escalating until it becomes a serious problem as it was with Trevor and Lucy. I'm reminded of an incident with one of my own children, when I narrowly missed falling into such a trap myself.

One evening as I was getting ready to leave for an important Family Life meeting in Seattle, nine-year-old Mike petulantly announced that he didn't want me to go. I explained that it was my job and that I had to be there. Dissatisfied with my reply, Mike followed me into the bathroom where I was applying fresh makeup.

"If you go," he told me, "I'll have an asthma attack."

A jolt of fear zapped my heart. I remembered the terrifying attacks he suffered as a small child. I remembered the long nights I sat holding him in my arms, listening to the damp hiss of the vaporizer, to his strangled breathing, willing the dragging minutes to pass and for the medication to take hold and bring relief. I remembered the stories I told, the soft songs I sang, hiding my fear, as I tried to help him relax as the lone, dark hours drained away.

Remembering all of this, I took a quick mental inventory of my son's present health. After three years of treatment, except for an occasional slight wheezing, readily controlled by a pill, Mike was no longer asthmatic — hadn't been for at least three years. He was, in fact, a healthy, athletic boy. At this moment the pollen season was over and he didn't have a cold. I could see no reason why he should have an asthma attack.

Startled, frightened as I was by the threat, I couldn't allow Mike to think that he could bring on an asthma attack at will, because in some cases it can happen. Nor could I allow him to believe that he could use the possibility of an attack as a weapon against me. For his own sake, I couldn't allow him to manipulate me in this way. Hardening my heart, I continued to apply my lipstick.

"I don't think you will have an attack." I told him in a calm, offhand voice. "If you do, take a pill. You know where they are."

Mike refrained from further protest — I kissed him good-bye and left for the meeting. It would be a lie to say that I didn't worry about Mike. The fact that the children were at home with their father who was perfectly capable of dealing with any emergency, failed to comfort me, and I fretted through the entire meeting. When I returned home at ten-thirty that night, the children were asleep in their beds. Mike was fine. There had been no asthma attack.

Trevor's story was never written up as a case study because the problem was so readily resolved and neither Daphne nor I were available to take sufficiently accurate data to make it a serious research project. Nevertheless it was an interesting learning experience and undoubtedly we both gained fresh insights into the dynamics of manipulative behaviors.

Chapter Six
Fircrest

I stood by a window watching the approach of an adolescent boy who appeared suddenly on the winding road leading to the school house. The boy was dancing, moving slowly in wide circles, his arms spread like wings. His wheat-stubble hair glinted in the sunlight. There was a brightness, a radiance about him, a young animal strength as he spiraled towards me, graceful and strong, unencumbered as a leaf twirling down from a tree — a yellow leaf against the cloudless blue of an August sky. Peter Pan, I thought of him, the dancing boy who did not hear and could not speak.

"Here comes Brian," I spoke to Claire, the teacher who was sorting books at the other end of the classroom.

"Brian?" She shrugged in surprise and turned to the door as he floated into the room.

"School?" Brian signed with his fingers.

"No," Claire signed back. "No more school. Later. Not now."

"Want school!" Brian signed emphatically and sat down at his desk.

"Holiday. Vacation. No more school." Claire gestured with equal emphasis. She sorted through her stack of books and papers and handed him a primer and a math work book.

Brian smiled. "Work?"

"Yes, work. Work at home."

Placing a hand on his shoulder, Claire guided Brian out the door. Clutching his books Brian leaped off the stoop and began dancing his way back to the residence hall.

It was August 1967. Less than three months before I was invited to develop a pilot educational program for forty residents at Fircrest, a state school for children and adults with developmental disabilities, located within the Seattle city limits. Two teachers, an audiologist and a psychologist were assigned to help me with the project.

As I accepted this summer assignment, I recalled my first day at the Rainier State School. I remembered how I cringed at what I saw, and how the first seeds of hope for the future of the children who were imprisoned, not only within the boundaries of that institution but within the prisons of their imperfect minds and bodies as well, took root within my heart. Now, barely two years later, I was back in a similar environment, not as a raw recruit, but as a champion, commissioned with the task of establishing the first academic program at Fircrest, and of proving once again what Dr. Bijou had proved to me: academic learning is possible even among those who are traditionally considered to be incapable of such achievement.

Twenty-three boys, and seventeen girls, ranging in age from nine to nineteen were enrolled in the Pilot Program. Their average I.Q. (intelligence quotient score as measured on the Standford Binet) was 26, as compared to the average score of 100 for the normal population. There were many problems and many different disabilities. There were brain-damaged, deaf, emotionally disturbed children, and children with Down syndrome. Some were hyperactive, destructive and aggressive. Others were silent, lethargic, withdrawn.

Seven of our students were able to speak in sentences of two or three words. A few more had a vocabulary of five to six words. The majority, however, had no expressive language whatsoever. Never in my life had I been faced with such a diverse group with so many seemingly insurmountable problems. As the first day of school approached, I became increasingly nervous. All of my training and experience had focused on working with preschool children. Now I would have to deal with school-age pupils, adolescents and young adults with severe disabilities. Envisioning a mob of forty disruptive and possibly aggressive individuals crowding into a single room, filled me with dismay. *How would I manage?* I wondered. *Would I be able to maintain control, avoid chaos?* Fortunately I was not alone. I was grateful for my staff and the fact that the two teachers, Margo and Claire, had taught in public school special education classes. I knew that I could rely on their support. Nevertheless I was in charge, and it was up to me to get the program off to a smooth start and to assure the attainment of our goals.

In order to accommodate forty pupils in a room designed for twelve, I divided the day into four ninety minute periods, with eight to twelve pupils in attendance at any one time. Tall cabinets and shelves separated the square, well-lit classroom into work areas where one teacher could supervise three to four pupils at a time.

On the first day of school we assessed the children on a number of tasks that were listed on a continuum, from sitting to attending, from scribbling to writing, from color and object recognition to reading and counting. A point was awarded each correct answer. Thirty six points equalled a perfect score. Following the assessment the children were grouped according to ability and readiness for designated tasks and assigned to either Claire, Margo or myself. Twenty-two subjects who scored between 0 and 9 on the test, and who had high rates of inappropriate behaviors were placed in a behavior modification program. The focus of this program was to teach the children to sit quietly in class, to make eye contact with the teacher, to imitate, to comply with routines and directions, and finally to learn how to work with basic manipulative materials such as blocks, puzzles and pegs.

Eight children were ready to begin a preacademic program. In this class the pupils learned how to match and discriminate colors, geometric shapes, pictures, numerals and letters of the alphabet. Imitation and language training such as I had done with Lucy were also a part of this curriculum.

Ten remaining children who scored well on the pretest entered an academic program. The children received instruction in reading, writing and arithmetic. Beginning with the simple matching of words to words, and words to pictures, the reading program progressed to reading from a pre-primer. Beginning with scribbling, joining dots and tracing, the writing program progressed to the printing of letters, words and numbers.

Mathematical concepts began with number recognition and sequencing to equating numbers to objects. Extreme disruptive behaviors such as destruction of materials, screaming, hitting, biting or self-mutilation such as head-banging were eliminated by withdrawing teacher attention or by the removing the troublemaker to a small empty room adjoining the classroom. All correct responses and behaviors were generously rewarded with food, tokens and/or praise. Throughout the program the emphasis was on enthusiastic teacher response to all desirable behaviors. At the end of our project, eight weeks after its inauguration, we reassessed our pupils. The results were gratifying. Twenty four pupils were now in the academic program. Fifteen were working at the preacademic level. One child left school due to illness. Not a single subject remained in the behavior modification program, each had advanced to a higher level. Except for a few minor incidents, our work progressed with remarkable smoothness. To this day I value the support of my staff and the rapport that was established between us, and I remember our pupils with great affection, some of whom remain in my mind with particular vividness.

JERRY

Jerry was a round-faced, freckled, redheaded nine-year-old boy. Jerry was in the behavior modification program, and I was his teacher. Jerry ran. It seemed impossible to contain him. Holding his hand was futile. Slippery as an eel, he broke loose and tore through the classroom, knocking over chairs, sweeping papers off desks, to dash headlong down the hall and out into the street. Not only did Jerry run and knock things down, he chewed things. Rather he devoured things, paper, wooden pencils and pegs, everything. One day after I managed to restrain Jerry by wedging him into a corner, barring his escape with a desk, I placed a box of small wooden pegs in front of him. Quick as a viper his hand darted out. He snatched up a handful of pegs and stuffed them into his mouth, grinding them up like a pencil-sharpener. Horrified, at the risk of losing a finger, I pried his mouth open and scooped out the splintered wood.

I worked with Jerry for three weeks. By the end of that time, the running had been brought under control. Jerry learned to walk by my side or to stay in line with his peers. He also learned to remain seated in his chair and to fill a peg board with fifty pegs, taking them out of a box, one by one and placing them systematically into the holes in the board, and not in his mouth. At the end of the exercise, I gave him lots of praise and a small dish of ice cream. The process of teaching him how to place pegs correctly began with the routine of receiving one teaspoon of ice cream each time a peg was inserted into the board. Gradually I increased the number of pegs that had to be placed before he received a treat.

Regretfully, on the day that Jerry succeeded in attending long enough to fill the entire peg board, he became ill with Shegala. Shegala is a highly infectious form of diarrhea. His whole ward was placed under quarantine, and Jerry was compelled to drop out of school.[8]

TOM, DICK and HARRY

Two days after Claire had begun working with three seventeen-year-old youths in the behavior modification class, she came to me with a complaint.

"Something has to be done. It's impossible to work with those boys."

I knew what she meant. The weather had been unusually hot, and Claire's class met in the afternoon. By that time, after baking in the sun all day, our wooden building and classroom were imbued with heat. Open windows brought an occasional breath of fresh air, but it failed to dissipate the nauseatingly pungent body odors emanating from the boys.

"Yes," I agreed. "They need a course in personal hygiene."

The next day I brought three washcloths, three towels, a bar of deodorizing soap, a spray deodorant, and several clean shirts. I obtained these things from general supplies. Since the residents wore donated clothing that came from various charitable organizations, it was a simple matter to get the shirts as well as the towels and soap. On making my request to the Fircrest housekeeper, I was directed to a large basement room filled with bins of jumbled clothing and other articles. By rummaging through the bins I found everything that I needed.

When the boys arrived at school, Claire and I took them into the bathroom, told them to remove their smelly shirts and proceeded to teach them how to lather, rinse and dry their bodies, and how to apply the deodorant. Although the boys required a great deal of supervision, they responded with good humor, and were grinning with self-importance when they finally emerged from the bathroom, wearing clean shirts and smelling of Old Spice. This became a daily procedure, and eventually the young men learned how to keep clean and "deodorized" without our supervision.

SLUGGO

As it happens in all institutions, Fircrest had its share of violent, psychotic residents. These unfortunates were housed under heavy security in a separate building and were not generally seen by anyone not directly involved with their care. Among these isolated residents was a young man nicknamed Sluggo. Sluggo was famous for escaping the confines of his ward and for going on violent rampages, demolishing everything in his path.

One morning towards the end of my eight-week project at Fircrest, I arrived at school to find that our front door had been torn off its hinges. An old screen door was fitted in its place.

"What happened?" I asked the custodian who happened to be in the building.

"Sluggo went crazy mad again. Busted ten windows and kicked in your door."

"Is it going to be fixed?"

"They're making a new one in the shop, but it may take a while. Got to fix the windows first. All that broken glass, kids might get hurt."

I didn't argue and went inside to prepare for the first class period of the day.

Finally it was Friday afternoon again. Classes were over for the week, and everyone had gone home. I remained behind to water the plants. I had just filled a pitcher with water when the phone rang. It was the Fircrest school secretary.

"I was told to warn you," she said. "Sluggo got out. They're looking for him now. He may be heading your way."

"Thanks." I hung up, locked the screen door and glanced out the window. There was no one in sight, nevertheless I decided to hurry through my task and leave as quickly as I could.

A few minutes later I heard a terrific banging on the screen door and a howling like that of an enraged cougar. Glancing into the hallway, I saw the dark outline of a man, kicking and punching the fragile door. I still held a water-filled pitcher in my hand. Without thinking, I ran forward and flung the water in his face. For a brief instant our eyes locked through the screen. His dark eyes had the wide, startled look of someone jarred out of sleep, but his wet face was blank, washed clean of all rage and emotion. I felt a surge of pity for this wild, confused boy.

"Go home, Sluggo," I said in a firm, but not unkind voice, speaking as I would to a rambunctious puppy.

Shaking the water out of his shaggy head, he turned obediently and slouched away.

BRIAN

Brian, our dancing boy, was one of those whose progress had been the most remarkable. When we first met Brian, he was a robot who moved through space in a mechanical stupor. Like a zombie under the evil spell of a witch doctor, he neither reacted nor initiated, but did as he was told, unspeaking, withdrawn, his face unchanging, his eyes fixed on some distant spot. When Brian was an infant his parents were told that he was born profoundly retarded, incapable of any intelligent thought. As a result his parents abandoned him. Brian was institutionalized and forgotten. No one, it appeared, bothered to question this initial diagnosis until Claire began working with him in the Pilot Program. A mother with teenage sons of her own, Claire was drawn to this silent, frozen boy. Moreover, Brian's behavior reminded her of some of the deaf children she encountered in special education classes outside of Fircrest.

Claire decided to teach Brian sign language. She began by showing him pictures of familiar objects, signing and saying the words as she did so. Day after day Claire repeated the exercise; day after day, Brian watched passively, seemingly indifferent to what was going on. Then suddenly he came to life. I remember the morning it happened. Once again Claire was working with Brian, and once again there was no reaction from him. Undaunted, she showed him yet another picture. It was a picture of a jacket.

"Jacket," she said, signing the word.

Brian pushed back his chair, strode out to the coat rack in the hallway and, before anyone could follow him, returned carrying his wind breaker. He laid the jacket on the table next to the picture. He looked straight at Claire, his gray-blue eyes burned with fierce intensity — something smoldering within him had burst into flames.

"Jacket," repeated Claire, signing the letters.

Intently, laboriously Brian attempted to imitate her gesture.

"Yes, yes!" Claire exclaimed, tears misting her eyes. Clasping his fingers she guided them through the proper configuration.

The fire in his eyes spread to his face in a beautiful, spontaneous smile. Like a moth breaking out of its cocoon, Brian rose to his feet, raised his arms, spread them wide and turned in a slow, graceful circle. Fairy godmother Claire had broken the spell, the enchanted young prince was free.

From that moment Brian surged ahead, mastering everything that Claire placed before him, math, reading, writing, spelling. Brian may have been born profoundly deaf, but he was definitely not mentally retarded. Neglected for sixteen years, and still handicapped by his deafness, Brian had an enormous amount of catching up to do. By the time the program ended, however, Brian was well on his way.

Among other things, Claire taught him new math which deals with numbers in an abstract way, not very different from the basic approach to algebra. Claire wrote a problem on the blackboard. If a+b=c, and a=c-b, what does b equal? Picking up a piece of chalk, Brian confidently wrote the correct answer: b=c-a. The ease with which Brian grasped these new concepts filled me with awe and disbelief. Without a doubt Brian was a highly intelligent boy.

Even after the Pilot Program ended, Claire maintained contact with Brian. He was a frequent guest in her home, staying for days at a time. In the fall of that year Brian began attending public school classes for the deaf, although he still lived at Fircrest. A few years later I learned that Brian had left Fircrest and was living independently, earning his living as a dog groomer in a pet shop.

There were other success stories, perhaps not as dramatic as Brian's transformation, but equally gratifying in terms of individual achievement. There was, for example, Trisha. Trisha was an eleven-year-old girl with Down syndrome who had lived at Fircrest since infancy. A pleasing, docile child, with a speaking vocabulary of a few words, she was generally attentive and responsive to adult demands. Yet Trisha had none of the preacademic skills that children normally master in the first three or four years of life. With Trisha, as with the other children in the preacademic class, it was necessary to teach her how to work with puzzles and blocks and how to match and recognize colors, shapes and pictured objects.

Trisha learned quickly, progressing rapidly from color and picture recognition to words and letters. By the end of the eight-week project, Trisha was reading from a pre-primer and ready to tackle more advanced reading material.

Best of all, the end of the Pilot Program didn't signal an end to our efforts. On the contrary, the project became the springboard for a permanent school program at Fircrest. Moreover, after I left Fircrest to return to my work at the University, Margo and Claire remained to continue what we had started.

When the Fircrest school program resumed in September, Trisha was among the returning pupils. Three years later Trisha left Fircrest to live in a foster home and to continue her schooling in a special education class within the regular public school system. As an adult Trisha is living in a group home and working in a sheltered workshop.

Five years after the inauguration of the Pilot Program, the Fircrest school continued to operate with 170 children in attendance. When I collected this follow-up information, 38 pupils were enrolled at the behavior modification level; 58 were attending preacademic classes; 62 were doing academic work and 12 more were receiving vocational training. Seventeen additional residents were attending public schools or working in sheltered workshops. A hairline crack to the outside world had appeared in the solid wall of institutionalism.

Chapter Seven
Dennis*

Fall quarter began and I returned to my duties at DPL. Florence Harris congratulated me on what had been accomplished at Fircrest. Her words warmed me, but they failed to dispel the feeling of dismay that had tinged my sense of achievement from the day that the Pilot Program ended. Dominant in my mind was the rcalization that thc vcry skills wc taught at Fircrest to nine and fifteen-year-old pupils are acquired by normal children within the first three years of life.

What would happen, I asked myself, if we began teaching these basic developmental skills to handicapped infants at the same time that these abilities emerge in normal babies? Would not this early training enable the disabled child to profit from the experience, and to accelerate his development? As I pondered these questions I searched in my mind for a way that I could put these ideas into practice.

Today, fortunately, infant programs and infant learning are recognized as essential components within the field of special education. In 1967, however, infant learning was unknown and the very concept of such a thing was viewed with great skepticism. In my decision to seek out babies with obvious delays in order to begin a program of developmental acceleration, I would be striking out across untrodden terrain.

As I made my plans, I could foresee that my undertaking and any claims to success would be regarded with suspicion by medical and educational professionals. The belief that maturation would eventually overcome all developmental delays was firmly entrenched in their collective minds. I feared, and rightly so, I'm sure, that any progress made by infants who had obvious retardation, but no definite medical diagnosis of the problem, would be credited solely to maturation and not necessarily to the effectiveness of any program. Thus, I realized that I would have to begin my work with a group that could be unequivocally diagnosed as having identical, identifiable and irreversible problems. For these reasons, and for the following considerations, I decided to focus my initial efforts on babies with Down syndrome.

The incidence of Down syndrome is high. One baby out of every 1000 live births is so diagnosed. Down syndrome is recognizable at birth, and a blood test can readily prove or disprove the diagnosis.

Traditionally children with Down syndrome were considered to be severely retarded, and the majority were institutionalized at an early age. As a result of my experience with this population at Fircrest I doubted the validity of such pessimistic views, and I suspected that the myths and attitudes towards Down syndrome were based upon hearsay and misinformation.

Intrigued as I was by the ideas germinating in my mind, I was willing to wait, to bide my time, until a plan could be fully formulated. Then suddenly, the whole matter was taken out of my hands and I plunged into a current of events that was to carry me faster and farther than I had ever dreamed possible, shaping, changing my life, and bearing me and my future associates to worldwide, expanding horizons.

One morning shortly after I had returned to the University, I met Dennis. This blue-eyed, blond, curly-haired boy became the catalyst that changed the whole course of my life and the lives of all the children with Down syndrome that I was destined to meet.

Dennis was seven months old. He had been born with Down syndrome and also club feet. He appeared on the scene, his legs encased in hip-high plaster casts, riding on his mother's back in a backpack. His older brother was attending the Laboratory Preschool and Dennis happened to be accompanying his mother when she came to take the older boy home.

I saw Dennis, and suddenly everything that I had experienced and thought about since my weeks at Fircrest exploded in my mind with overwhelming urgency. I approached Dennis' mother, and without even considering any pros or cons, quickly outlined the kind of infant learning program that I would like to establish. As I explained that what I was proposing was unknown and untried, I tried to reassure her that I did know children and child development, and that my goal was to help her son attain developmental landmarks at a rate as close to normal as possible.

Dennis' mother was a young woman with blue eyes and straight, bobbed hair, as blond as her son's. She studied me in silence, her cerulean eyes holding mine. Then, she eased the backpack off her shoulders and lifted Dennis.

"Here he is," she said gravely and handed him to me.

From my first brief interview with Dennis, I could see that he was already behind in a number of areas. Hampered by the heavy casts on his legs, Dennis spent a major portion of the day reclining in an infant seat. Accustomed to leaning back in his chair, his vision focused on a point near the ceiling, he didn't know how to look at things directly in front of his eyes, even when they were offered to him. He didn't reach for, nor grasp toys in the manner of a normal seven-month-old, and he was unable to sit upright by himself, another skill most children attain by that age.

I worked with Dennis four days a week for twenty minutes each time his mother came to get the older brother after preschool. Dennis was a charming little boy who delighted me with his eagerness to perform, his happy smiles and his engaging enthusiasm as he mastered progressively difficult tasks. A month before his first birthday, the casts were removed. His legs were strong and straight, although he had yet to learn how to stand and bear weight on the soles of his newly corrected feet. In the weeks that followed, Dennis learned how to crawl, how to pull himself to a standing position, and how to take his first steps, holding on the furniture. Meanwhile, encouraged by Dennis' progress, his pediatrician, Dr. Connie MacDonald* referred five more newly born babies with Down syndrome to me.

As I worked with Dennis and the other infants, I began developing sets of procedures for attaining specific results. I discovered, for example, that several easily performed pull-to-sit exercises increased head, neck and trunk control. It is necessary for a child to acquire these skills in order to sit, stand and walk independently. Other activities that focused on developing eye-hand coordination, language, cognitive and self-help skills were also devised. Since at this time children with Down syndrome were not generally expected to attain head, neck and trunk control, sitting and walking abilities until their second, third or even fourth year of life, the rapid improvement shown by infants under my regime of exercises was encouraging and exciting.

Busy and happy though I was, deeply engrossed with the infants and the program that I was developing, I couldn't escape the acrid smoke of the spreading conflagration in Vietnam. My sons, like thousands of young men across the land, still faced the draft. By now Mike had graduated from the University and married a classmate; a lovely young woman who was as comfortable in an old pair of cutoff jeans hosing down a boat, as she was behind a desk, wearing a designer suit, Gucci shoes and pearl earrings. Mike and Carol were vacationing in Hawaii when Mike was called up for his physical. As we braced ourselves for the inevitable, Mike received word that an old injury made him unfit for military service. His A-1 status was changed to indefinite exemption.

One rainy afternoon, when Mike was five years old, he went to play with a friend who lived across the street. As the boys clattered down to a basement play room, Mike slipped and fell down the stair well, thirteen feet to a concrete floor. Not realizing the extent of possible injuries, our neighbor merely phoned to say that Mike had fallen and that he was returning home. The next minute I saw Mike staggering towards me, sobbing in a strange, high-pitched voice. As I rushed to embrace him, he vomited a pool of blood and collapsed in my arms. Cold with terror I carried him into the house and telephoned a doctor. X-rays revealed that Mike suffered a skull fracture and a concussion. After five anxious days Mike was pronounced out of danger and on the way to recovery. Subsequent tests showed, however, that although there was no brain damage, the fracture, which had occurred on the left side of his head, might permanently impair Mike's hearing in that ear.

Thus, this childhood accident that had caused such anxiety in the past, served to spare us even greater anxiety, if not the ultimate sorrow of losing a son in battle. As I thanked a merciful fate for this turn of events, I couldn't forget the slaughter of the war nor the men and women who had to endure its horrors. My heart ached for them and for their loved ones. Nor could I forget that our second son, Alex, would soon, in his turn be eligible for the draft.

Alex was now twenty-one. In a few weeks he would complete his senior year at the University. Upon graduation he would no longer enjoy student deferment. Meanwhile as the conflict in Vietnam escalated, so did the anti-war sentiments across the nation. No different from their peers in other institutions, the students at the University of Washington staged demonstrations. Together with his classmates Alex walked in a peace march across the I-5 Ship Canal Bridge, protesting the invasion of Cambodia. Nevertheless, Alex didn't burn his draft card, and if called, I knew that he would obey the summons. Fortunately that never came to pass, and the terrible bloodshed finally came to an end.

Against this background I continued my work with Dennis and other infants with Down syndrome. The children thrived and grew older. By the end of 1969 I realized that I would have to make a change in my professional life if the program were to succeed. Many of the infants were now toddlers and ready for preschool. Moreover, I had a waiting list of several babies whom I could no longer fit into my schedule. The program demanded a full time commitment. I needed regular classroom space and at least one assistant teacher. None of these was possible as long as I remained in my present position where I was paid for running a preschool for typical children, and not for working with devlopmentally delayed infants. The minutes I devoted to these children were snatched during lunch breaks and after hours. Although Florence Harris and our new director, Dr. Hal B. Robinson*, were tolerant, even supportive of my extra curricular activities, this arrangement couldn't continue indefinitely. My degree was in special education, my interest lay in working with disabled children. I didn't belong in the Department of Psychology where I was tolerated and perhaps valued, but where I could never advance beyond my status as head teacher and where my program for children with Down syndrome would never receive the recognition I hoped it deserved.

I approached Florence Harris and asked her advice. This kind, enthusiastic woman told me what I wanted to hear. It was time to move on. My experimental work with infants, she pointed out, had not gone unnoticed by certain Special Education faculty members. Among them were Dr. Charles H. Strother*, Dr. Norris Haring* and Dr. Alice H. Hayden*, three individuals in key positions at the newly opened Child Development and Mental Retardation Center, now renamed as the Center on Human Development and Disability (CHDD). The purpose of this center at the University of Washington is to provide training, service and research within a multi-disciplinary approach to child health, development and education. One of these disciplines, education, is housed in a separate adjoining facility, known as the Experimental Education Unit (EEU). The Unit is basically a school with classrooms serving mentally and developmentally retarded children of all ages. Within these classrooms, teachers and staff concentrate on developing innovative research based programs which can best serve the educational needs of these children. The classrooms are in a sense laboratories, testing fields for the development of model programs which, once tested and proven to be successful, can be transported and replicated in public school or institutional settings. At the time of which I write, Dr. Strother was director of CDMRC, Dr. Haring was director of EEU; Dr. Alice Hayden, the third member of this trio, directed the EEU preschool programs.

"Talk to these people," Florence Harris urged me. "I know for a fact they want you to join their academic staff."

Chapter Eight
Pitfalls and Plaudits

I followed Florence Harris's advice and with the coming of the New Year found myself installed at the Experimental Education Unit. Dr. Hayden, my immediate superior, and director of the preschool component at the Unit, had already established two classrooms for four-year-olds, who exhibited behavior and language deficits. The tenor of the times was changing. The child diagnosed as moderately retarded and who had been denied a public school education a few years ago, was no longer institutionalized. Society was beginning to accept these children and the government was ready to support university programs which promised to develop educational models for this population. This new acceptance, however, didn't as yet include the child with Down syndrome nor the concept of infant learning. All of this would happen later. First the educability of these children had to be established.

Welcomed aboard, I was given office space and a raise in salary, but neither a classroom nor official recognition for babies and toddlers with Down syndrome. I drifted for another full year, fulfilling a number of unrelated tasks. Mainly I conducted workshops and served as a resource teacher and consultant to Head Start and public school special education classes. Once again by snatching moments of free time and by seeking out available space wherever and whenever I could, I managed to continue my work with Dennis and his peers. Sustained by the hope that Dr. Hayden's vague promise to start a program for children with Down syndrome would be realized, I tried to curb my frustration and performed my various assignments as conscientiously as I could.

That hope was not in vain. Without my knowledge, Hayden applied for a grant on my behalf. By January 1971 funding was granted at federal and state levels and my dream of an early educational program for children with Down syndrome became a reality.

Alice Hayden was tall, big bosomed and some ten years older than I. Her appearance was noteworthy for its lack of color and style. She remains in my mind as a brownish-beige blur. Her overcoats were beige, her ill-fitting polyester pants-suits, beige or a diluted brown, like watery cocoa, matched her open-toed, canvas topped, wedge-heeled shoes. Even her hair, cut short and marcelled close to her head in a 1920s style was a faded, copper-brown, as were her almost nonexistent eyebrows and lashes. Her eyes, the color of withered leaves, peered intently through a pair of rimless glasses.

Except for a smudge of pink across thin lips and a dusting of white powder, she wore no makeup. Beneath its coating of talc, her face looked flat and spongy, like a floured circle of dough. In contrast to this overall blandness, Dr. Hayden favored chunky earrings and strands of beads, and her hands, her best feature, were beautifully groomed. Her fingers were long and slender, the manicured nails, glossy with colorless enamel.

On her right hand, she wore a single ring, a large, brilliantly green jade stone, set in an oval gold setting.

Hayden's personal life was a mystery. There was no visible family and she lived alone in one half of a brick duplex which she owned. Dr. Hayden didn't drive. A close friend and companion, an unmarried, middle-aged teacher who occupied the second half of the building, drove her back and forth to work every day.

I soon learned that Dr. Hayden's bland appearance was deceptive. By nature she was an abrasive woman, quick to take umbrage and quick to strike with sharp, belittling retorts. Along with this she had a keen mind and a prodigious memory for names, dates and numbers. Lacking this talent for trivia, I was often at a disadvantage.

On paper Hayden expressed herself with aplomb. She wrote endless reports and persuasive grant proposals, swinging through the ropes of grantsmanship with the flair of a trapeze artist. When it came to verbal communication this artistry failed her. She spoke in vague, disjointed sentences. Studding her words with unfamiliar names, acronyms, and confusing figures she leaped from one drifting thought to another like Eliza among the ice floes. One colleague ventured that Dr. Hayden must be a latent stutterer. Perhaps. Whatever the reason, it was often painful to listen to her presentations. Yet she was highly esteemed and had earned the reputation of being so advanced in knowledge, so eminently superior to the members of her audiences that only the most erudite could hope to comprehend her incomprehensible lectures. In later years, students taking her seminars frequently came to me for clarification.

Working for Hayden, I discovered, was like walking through a dark cellar full of cobwebs and hidden dangers. Never explicit, never direct in her requests, names and acronyms dropping like booby-traps, I groped through her words as I would through a mine field or through a net of spiderwebs, seeking some small clue to guide me in the right direction. Questions irritated her, and if I failed to immediately recognize who J.P. or Marty, Helen or Carl might be, and their connection to HEW, JRP, WESTAR or to some other government agency, she was scathing in her disdain.

One Wednesday afternoon, in my second year at the Unit, Hayden summoned me into her office.

"G.B. needs a report for NDN by Friday morning," she announced.

Report? G.B.? NDN? I was in the cellar again.

"Ah, yes, G.B., of course," stalling for time, I tried to circle my way through the swathing words. "A report, yes, on what topic, did he say?"

"He!" Her yellow eyes snapped at me behind the rimless glasses. "Since when is Gertrude Beatrice Bundhiemer a man!"

Ouch! I had stubbed my toe again.

Friday morning I took the finished report to Hayden's office. Uncertain about what was expected of me, but assuming that an update on our new program for children with Down syndrome might suffice, I compiled some figures, reviewed current data on individual and group progress, prepared a few graphs, outlined future objectives, and wrapped everything together with a two paragraph summary. The result was a ten-page manuscript which was typed and ready for me when I returned to work on Friday.

Hunched down in a chair, her glasses lying on the desk, Hayden was peering at a journal article through a magnifying glass.

I approached tentatively. "Here's the report, Dr. Hayden."

She nodded curtly, without raising her head. This seeming coldness chilled me. Was I in the wrong again? I worked extra hours on the report and believed that I deserved better acknowledgment. I attempted to soften the moment.

"I had some good data to report. I hope Gertrude Bundhiemer approves."

"G.B. has nothing to do with this," Hayden muttered irritably, eyes glued on the page. "She's sending it on to Chris!"

Chris? Who was he? She?

"Yes, of course." I murmured leaving hurriedly.

Poor woman, I thought to myself, so myopic she is practically blind. I decided to forgive her.

Sometimes, however, it was harder to overlook her rudeness. On one occasion both Hayden and I were speakers at a large conference held at the University of Illinois. As I stepped up to the podium, I saw Hayden sitting in the front row. I smiled at my audience, some three hundred students and high-ranking educators, and included her in my smile. Asked to speak on our innovative program for children with Down syndrome, I began with a description of the setting. After describing the classroom, I mentioned the outdoor area where the children engaged in gross motor activities.

"Just before juice time the children are taken to the play court," I said.

"Not play court," Hayden corrected me loudly and scornfully from her front row seat, "outdoor classroom, if you please!"

"Outdoor classroom," I parroted, humoring her, and somehow managing to keep my poise. Still angry, and although I had heard her heckle colleagues in the same manner, blood rushed to my cheeks. In later years I learned to ignore her rudeness, but it rankled, just the same.

Nevertheless, despite her irritability, vagueness and persnicketiness, I became fond of Alice Hayden. She was a complex, unpredictable woman, and I never fully understood her, but I prized her ability, her willingness to accept new ideas and her readiness to seize opportunities as she did when I proposed my fledgling Down syndrome program to her. I valued her support and I fully appreciated the funding she obtained on my behalf. Most of all I admired and respected her for giving me a carte blanche when it came to running the program and to setting increasingly challenging goals as the pupils progressed from preschool to kindergarten and on to public school.

"I think children with Down syndrome can learn to read," I told Hayden after Dennis and several other four-year-olds in the advanced preschool had acquired the necessary pre-reading skills. "I'd like to start a reading program."

"Wonderful!" exclaimed Dr. Hayden. "Go right ahead."

As I hoped the children did learn how to read, write, count and speak. Dennis also learned these subjects, but he spoke in unintelligible croaks and grunts. Sadly we learned, that our smiling, gentle, flaxen-haired Dennis, was growing progressively deaf.

I was destined to remain at the Experimental Education Unit for the next twelve years. These were busy, productive years. By 1974 the program had expanded from one classroom with eleven pupils to five with an enrollment of over fifty children. Assuming the role of coordinator, I left the classroom to supervise a staff of five head teachers and an equal number of practicum student teacher aides. As the program grew so did our visibility and renown. Telephone calls and mail requesting information and personal appearances at meetings and workshops as well as letters from parents seeking comfort, advice and answers to questions became a daily occurrence. In addition to ongoing administrative duties, I answered all letters, wrote and published articles and reports, developed slide shows and video tape presentations, lectured at local and national conferences and assisted parent groups, outside of Seattle, to establish their own programs for developmentally delayed youngsters. This burden of work might have become overwhelming were it not for my excellent, handpicked staff and their wholehearted dedication to the goals of our endeavor. Patricia Oelwein* and Patsy Love* two of my wonderful head teachers became the backbone of the program and my dearest friends. Patsy retired shortly after I did in 1982, but Patricia Oelwein is still at the University of Washington carrying on the work I began twenty-six years ago.

Every summer from the onset of the program my staff and I conducted a three-week workshop on Down syndrome and special education. University credit was available to the participants and the workshops became very popular. Parents, teachers and students, not only from nearly every state in the Union, but from all over the world flocked to our classes. Mingling with the Americans, men and women from Japan, Mexico, Spain, Guatemala, Canada, Indonesia, Hong Kong and Australia filled the auditorium. Many parents from the States as well as from foreign countries brought their disabled babies and children seeking first hand information on how to deal with individual problems. It was gratifying to help these people and exciting to find so many different cultures and nationalities banded together by mutual concerns.

At the end of the workshop, it became a custom for me to invite foreign and out of state visitors to a buffet dinner at our home. One time as we sat on the patio sipping wine, after a meal of cold poached salmon, potato salad, and blueberry cobbler, I turned to the group and asked how many different languages were spoken there, that evening.

"I speak Korean," volunteered a statuesque Asian woman.

"French," replied a nun from Montreal.

"Italiano," smiled a young doctor from Naples.

"Japanese," giggled petite Noriko.

"Russian," I chimed in.

"Spanish," chorused a mixed group of parents and teachers, from Madrid, Barcelona, Mexico and Guatemala.

"Malaysian," offered Lily, a brown-skinned neurologist from Jakarta.

There was a pause, and then a pert, dark-haired, blue-eyed teacher from Georgia spoke up.

"And I," she drawled softly, "speak South'rn."

In 1974, all of the programs that received federal grants under The Handicapped Children's Early Assistance Act of 1968, including our program for children with Down syndrome, were evaluated by the Joint Review and Dissemination Panel for the Bureau of Education for Handicapped Children, U.S. Department of Health Education and Welfare. Based upon our data and the children's exceptional progress, our program for Children with Down syndrome was one of the first of seven innovative programs to be validated by this committee as an exemplary program worthy of replication and adaptation by schools and centers across the nation. This was a big honor and assured continued funding for the program.

Early in 1975 I went to North Ryde, an area some twenty miles north of Sydney, Australia. The purpose of my visit was to train teachers and to establish a replication of the Down syndrome program at the University of MacQuarie. During my three weeks at MacQuarie I was assisted by Moira Pieterse*, a charming Australian woman, an experienced teacher with a Master's Degree in Special Education and the mother of six children. As we laid the groundwork for the program, Moira and I became good friends. Our work progressed swiftly and smoothly. Children were enrolled and assessed. Equipment and materials were purchased and arranged in an empty classroom. Several university students, majoring in special education were selected and assigned as teacher trainees. Before I left, Patricia Oelwein, as the most skilled teacher at the Experimental Education Unit, came to take my place. Patricia was accompanied by her husband and two children. Her job was to supervise the new program for the next two months. When it was time for the Oelweins to return to Seattle, yet another teacher from the University of Washington Down syndrome program travelled to Australia to continue the work we began. Kristin Nichols* and her husband, Peter, remained in Australia, until the following June, at which time, the students training in the classroom received their degrees and were sufficiently prepared to carry on the program.

With Kristin's departure, Moira Pieterse became the coordinator and supervisor of the program. This experiment was a success. Under Moira's dedicated guidance the MacQuarie program flourished, and has in its turn, been replicated within Australia, in several South Asian countries including Hong Kong, and in a number of European cities as well.

My travels continued. Over the years I made several trips to Spain, Japan, Canada and Mexico. Everywhere I went I conducted workshops and helped establish replications of our model. At other times I attended conferences and gave presentations in Scotland, England, Hong Kong and Jakarta. This interest in my work was exceedingly gratifying, as was the fact that my book *Time to Begin* was translated into German and Japanese and published in these countries. A few years later *Advances in Down syndrome*, a book which Patricia Oelwein and I co-edited, was also translated and published in Japan.

By the end of the decade we were serving over a hundred children with Down syndrome, half of this number were still attending classes at EEU, the remaining pupils were graduates of the program and were now attending classes within the public school system. Meanwhile replications of our model were springing up nationwide, from Alaska to Florida. Committed to giving technical assistance to these replication sites, increasingly our work, Patricia Oelwein's and mine, focused on serving these offshoots of our model, and nearly every week one of us would be hurrying to the airport to catch a flight to Lubbock, Anchorage or Miami.

These were indeed, busy, exciting, gratifying years. Our pupils forged ahead, surpassing all of our expectations and revealing as yet untapped potentials. Doctors Hayden and Haring became increasingly enthusiastic about the program. Travelling around the country as VIPs do, they lauded *their* remarkable program for children with Down syndrome. At times I wished that they would give me and my staff a personal pat on the back and some credit for the success of our endeavor, but that never happened. Nevertheless the plaudits that I received from other sources, helped to compensate for the pitfalls I encountered in my daily dealings with Alice Hayden.

Chapter Nine
Home Visit

Polly Stokes was a sturdy, slightly overweight four-year-old, a newcomer who had entered the program for Down syndrome children midterm that fall. Thick brown hair, cut in a Dutch bob framed a lively round face and accented a pair of mischievous brown eyes. A bright, active child, Polly obviously enjoyed school and seemed able and willing to meet our expectations. Pleased with Polly's progress, we were surprised when Mrs. Stokes began complaining about her child's behavior at home.

"She's impossible, absolutely, impossible ... so difficult to manage," Helen Stokes confessed, reddening with embarrassment.

After questioning Mrs. Stokes further, we made a number of helpful suggestions, but to no avail. The complaints continued and Mrs. Stokes looked increasingly distraught.

"You have no idea what Polly's like at home. She gets into everything. I simply can't watch her all the time!" she insisted wearily.

Finally I suggested a home visit, explaining that after seeing the home situation I might be in a better position to offer a solution to the problem. We agreed on a Saturday morning. I would come after breakfast and stay through the lunch hour.

I arrived around 9:30 A.M. The Stokes lived in a deteriorating residential neighborhood. I walked through a fallen gate, across a cracked concrete walk, matted with weeds, and up a set of sagging steps to a weather-beaten, ramshackled two-storied house. Polly opened the door. She was in a nightgown, barefooted. She carried a half eaten piece of toast, and her face was smeared with crumbs and jelly. The front room was bare and shabby, furnished with a worn gray rug, a badly battered couch, a TV, and two chests of drawers. One was tied with a rope, and the other turned to face the wall. A few tinker-toy pieces and a couple of tattered picture books lay on the floor.

Helen Stokes, a tall, large-boned woman, with a plain, but not unattractive face, came to meet me. She was wearing a faded flannel robe, her long, graying hair was pulled back in a careless knot. She gave an apologetic shrug and explained that the front room was purposely bare. This was where they kept Polly away from the rest of the house.

"Polly likes to jump on the couch and watch TV," she said, adding that the rope around the chest was her husband's idea. He didn't want Polly messing around in the drawers. The other chest faced the wall for the same reason.

Albert Stokes was not at home. He had been unemployed for over a year, and they had been on welfare for several months. However, he was working at last, as an orderly in a hospital. He worked the early morning shift and would return by lunchtime.

We went into the dining room which was furnished with odds and ends of discarded furniture. There were dirty dishes on the table and Polly's unfinished breakfast of dry cereal and milk. Mrs. Stokes cleared a spot at the table and poured two cups of tea. We sat down to talk. Behind the hooked door to the front room I could hear Polly jumping on the couch. The television was on full blast. Presently there was a commotion. Ann, the younger of Polly's two teenaged sisters, came clattering down the stairs from the upper story. She was in her pajamas. She stormed into the front room and snapped off the TV. Polly protested, screaming. Mrs. Stokes intervened. I could hear her cajoling Ann and trying to comfort Polly.

Peace was restored. The TV was turned on again, but with less volume. Ann went into the kitchen. Helen Stokes and I resumed our conversation. She began telling me how hard it was for her to manage her two daughters and Polly. Mr. Stokes was no help. Suddenly there was a crash in the kitchen, followed by shrieks and screams from Ann. Mrs. Stokes and I rushed to investigate. Polly had "escaped" from the front room and had knocked over an open canister of sugar. As I surveyed the mess, and began helping Mrs. Stokes clean up, I was appalled at the disorder in the kitchen. All the cupboard doors were open and all of the counters were cluttered with dishes and staples that had apparently been taken off the shelves and never replaced. Lids were off jars and bottles, and in addition to the sugar that was now on the floor, there was also a trail of spilled dry cereal and other edibles. The sugar was probably also standing open, within easy reach of Polly's prying fingers. Anyone could see that the clutter in the kitchen had not been created by Polly, but with so many things within reach, I could see why Polly was always getting into trouble.

About this time, Mary, the oldest daughter, appeared. She was dressed in a shirt and jeans, ready to go to work. She worked as a waitress in a drive-in. She was an attractive girl of about seventeen, but at this moment her face was flushed. She darted at Polly and began shaking and scolding her. Polly, it seemed, had dumped Mary's bath salts into the toilet. Polly, who had been sitting on the floor, calmly stuffing Cheerio bits into her mouth and licking her sugary fingers, began to sob.

"Oh, Mary, leave her alone! She's just a baby!" The mother exclaimed. She reached for Polly and carried her out of the room. Sitting on a chair in the dining room, she held and rocked Polly. It looked as if she too was ready to cry.

"Let's help your mother clean this up," I said to the two girls who were still in the kitchen.

"This place is a pig pen!" Mary snapped. She snatched up a jacket that had fallen to the floor and stomped out the back door.

Ann went into the dining room and held out her arms to Polly.

"I'll play with her," she said kindly.

Polly slipped off her mother's lap and took Ann by the hand. A look of pride came over Mrs. Stokes' face.

"Ann can be very good with Polly, but she does get irritated. They all do."

A short time later Ann came out to the front room announcing that she had to shampoo her hair. She had left the room, leaving Polly locked behind. Polly began to whine. I glanced at my wrist watch, it was almost eleven o'clock.

Mrs. Stokes stirred. "I'd better take Polly to the bathroom." She pushed herself away from the table reluctantly. I urged her to attend to anything that she had to do, and not to let me interfere.

"I'll just take Polly upstairs," she replied.

When Mrs. Stokes returned she had changed into a pair of pants and a sweater. Polly was still in her nightgown, but she was carrying an armful of clothing.

"I'll help Polly get dressed," I volunteered, reaching for the child.

Mrs. Stokes thanked me and began clearing the table in a desultory manner. She seemed tired. Except for the floor which I had swept, the kitchen was still in shambles. I could hear Mrs. Stokes moving about, rattling utensils.

Polly squirmed and fussed as I tried to dress her. I ignored her fussing and began playing a game with her, pointing to and naming parts of her body. I took her toes and played "This little piggy went to market." Polly quieted down, giggled and repeated some of the words. As I pulled off her nightgown I saw that her buttocks were raw with diaper rash. Although toilet trained during the day, it was obvious that Polly wore a diaper at night. I made a mental note to ask her mother about this and also to speak to our school nurse.

After Polly was dressed I made the mistake of leaving her alone while I joined Mrs. Stokes in the kitchen. The moment my back was turned Polly bolted upstairs. Mrs. Stokes dropped what she was doing and ran after her. I heard the sounds of a struggle and Polly screaming in a tantrum. Finally, her face red and her hair dishevelled Helen Stokes returned, half dragging, half carrying Polly down the stairs. Polly was screaming and struggling. Mrs. Stokes thrust her into the front room and bolted the door. Polly continued to howl and hammer on the door.

"You see, I can't leave her for a minute! We have to watch her like a hawk. The moment my back is turned she gets into something!" her mother apologized.

"Why did she dash upstairs?"

"Oh, she wants to get into her sisters' room. Ann has a collection of Barbie dolls from the time that she was a little girl, and Polly just loves to get her hands on them. She also likes to play with Mary's cosmetics."

Polly had become quiet again. The TV was on, and Polly was jumping on the couch.

The back door slammed. Mrs. Stokes ran a hand over her hair. "That's my husband, he'll be wanting his lunch."

She went into the kitchen and I heard a murmur of voices. Albert Stokes came into the dining room and greeted me heartily. I had met him before. He was an aging, bushy haired, bearded man, who wore a cotton Mexican shirt and love beads. For a few minutes he talked expansively about how smart Polly was. Mrs. Stokes served him a bowl of soup and a sandwich. She said Polly would eat later.

I excused myself saying that I would look at a book with Polly while he ate. I went into the front room and as I sat down with the book Polly snuggled up to me. I deliberately left the door between the front room and the rest of the house ajar.

Mr. Stokes ate alone, reading a newspaper. His wife had disappeared. Ann came back, her hair in rollers. She said something to her father and he muttered a reply. Ann went into the kitchen and came out again carrying a sandwich and a can of pop. Presently I heard her in the hall talking to someone on the telephone.

Mrs. Stokes came out of the basement, carrying a basket of laundry. Mr. Stokes wanted some coffee; she brought it to him. It was almost 12:30. Mrs. Stokes said it was time for Polly's lunch. I said it was time to leave. Mr. Stokes got up from the table stretching. He had been at work since five that morning and he was going to take a nap. He told his wife he didn't want any noise. He said good-bye to me in a friendly manner and went upstairs. As I left I told Mrs. Stokes that I would arrange to talk to her later about how we could help her with Polly. Mrs. Stokes thanked me and said it was kind of me to come. She smiled. I saw that her teeth were pitted with cavities.

I left feeling very sad. My heart ached for Helen Stokes and for Polly. This family was under a great deal of stress. New arrivals from another state, they not only had to cope with the problems of relocation, they were also faced with the hardships of unemployment and downright poverty. One could easily understand the frustration and anger of the two teenaged girls, compounded by poverty, deprivation and the added impact of a troublesome sibling.

Obviously Mrs. Stokes was overwhelmed by the responsibilities of managing the household and keeping peace between her daughters. Whether she had always been a disorganized housekeeper or whether the disorder in the kitchen was a symptom of her present distress I was unable to say. Still, in spite of such shortcomings, Mrs. Stokes was the one who was shouldering the major part of the burden. Later I learned how great that burden really was. Four years before Polly's birth, Helen Stokes reached a momentous decision. She finally summoned enough courage to abandon a faltering, incompatible marriage and to seek a better life for herself and her two daughters. She left Albert, rented a small apartment for herself and the girls and got a job at a general store that sold hay and grain. Born and raised on a small farm in Kansas, Helen Stokes was in her element among the farm tools and harness, the fragrant bales of alfalfa and the clean robust smell of grain. For the first time in many years Helen Stokes was happy, full of vigor and hope for the future. But her freedom was short-lived. Within two months she could no longer deny the inevitable. After a hiatus of more than ten years, at age forty-two, she was incredibly, incomprehensibly, tragically pregnant. Helen returned to Albert; endured a hard, debilitating pregnancy and gave birth to Polly, a baby she didn't want, an unwanted baby with Down syndrome.

Polly was not abused physically, but emotionally she was sadly deprived. Her mother was not unkind, but it appeared to me that the bonding that takes place between mother and infant at birth, so crucial to a child's subsequent development, never occurred between Polly and her mother. Denied this supportive warmth, Polly became an irritating foreign presence in a hostile environment.

Superficially jovial, speaking expansively of his retarded daughter, Albert Stokes seemed in reality to be an alienated man who failed as a husband, a father and as a provider, for he never succeeded in holding a permanent job. Ann, the gentler of the two older sisters, was fickle in her attention to Polly, and she too showed signs of isolating herself from the family. Helen found herself caught in the middle with Polly on one side, her husband and the older girls on the other. It might appear that she was protecting them from Polly, and at the same time intervening and protecting Polly from them. In reality, however, Mrs. Stokes was shutting Polly out emotionally, as effectively as she was shutting her out physically behind the locked door — making it impossible for Polly to become assimilated into the family unit.

In trying to remedy this situation, I began by arranging for Polly to be out of the home for more than the two hours that she spent in preschool. This was achieved by enrolling Polly in Head Start. Polly was indeed a bright child with a great deal of natural curiosity and initiative. It was important for her to be constructively occupied. From what I had seen there was little of this available to her at home. Much of her disruptive behavior was the result of boredom, inactivity and loneliness. For the next two years, Polly attended both the Down syndrome program and Head Start until she entered first grade in a public school which served typical as well as developmentally delayed children.

I had hoped that attendance in Head Start would lessen the impact of her presence at home, and that her family would begin seeing Polly in a more positive light, but this didn't happen. Although Polly did well at school and caused few problems she continued to be disruptive and destructive at home. The older she became the more her sisters resented her, and the more difficult it became for Mrs. Stokes to control her. Through mischief and violence Polly continued to seek and gain the attention her parents had never been able to give her through love. Regretfully the Stokes were not ready or able to implement the parenting and behavior management skills that we tried to teach them.

When Polly turned sixteen, she was placed in a group home. A group home is a residence for small numbers of developmentally disabled teens and adults who for one reason or another are unable to remain with their families. The goal of the group home is to provide a homelike environment within the community, and to serve as a stepping stone to greater independence if and when an individual is ready to meet that challenge. By now, Polly is an adult. I don't know where she is or what she is doing. Mary and Ann are living their own lives. Helen Stokes is working at a well-paying job. She and Mr. Stokes are still together.

Chapter Ten
Diagnoses

The morning mail brought a letter from Macon, Georgia. I recognized the handwriting and sighed as I slit the envelope. I sighed not with annoyance but in sympathy for the writer. Barbara Thomas and I had been corresponding for several months. Her story was not unique and one that I had encountered many times. A premature baby with Down syndrome, her daughter, Lori, was a frail child, beset with health problems. In addition to a congenital heart murmur, she was exceedingly susceptible to colds, ear and bronchial infections, stomach upsets and pneumonia. In her brief life Lori had already been hospitalized five times. Barbara's letters were the continual outpourings of a despairing mother.

"What can I do?" she had written in one of her previous letters. "Lori has a fever again. How can I help her? I can't bear to see her so sick. Why can't the doctors keep her well? Surely there is something they can do! Why isn't she gaining weight?"

Unable to make specific recommendations sight unseen, I tried to respond as realistically and sympathetically as I could. "All premature infants, even normal babies, are at risk," I told her. "They need time to catch up. Keep her active, but avoid fatigue, feed her small amounts of nourishing food at frequent intervals. Look for another doctor," I counselled.

"Why isn't Lori sitting by herself?" Barbara questioned me in another letter. "She had her first birthday six months ago. My boys walked at twelve months!"

Although there were no early intervention programs for children with Down syndrome where they lived, there was a developmental center for generally disabled youngsters.

"Lori may need physical therapy," I wrote in reply to her query. "Take her to the developmental center."

Predictably, this day's letter brought new concerns.

"Lori has been receiving physical therapy three days a week for two months, and she still isn't sitting," I read. "She'll sit alone for a minute or two and then she falls over. The therapist says she's just lazy. Why should Lori be lazy? Why does she cry so much? She cries, whines, actually, nearly all the time. Her teacher, Miss Holcomb, says she's spoiled. I can't believe this is true. Even a spoiled baby wouldn't cry *all* the time. My new doctor tells me to ignore her. He claims all children with Down syndrome are fussy. Is that so? You told me that babies with Down syndrome are very much like any other infants. Something must be wrong, but what? Why doesn't someone tell me?"

As I pondered over these new developments, the phone rang. It was Barbara, calling me long distance.

"Val!" She sounded excited. "I have wonderful news. You can come to Macon!"

"I can?"

"Yes! The Developmental Center will sponsor you if you come here to give a workshop. Will you do it? Please say that you will, then you can see Lori and tell me what's wrong!"

"I'll come, and I'll see Lori, but I can't promise any answers," I told her.

"Don't say that! You're my last hope. You've worked with so many Down's kids, surely you can help me!"

"Well," I conceded, "perhaps I will notice something that has been overlooked. I agree with you, constant crying isn't normal under any circumstances." I turned to my calendar. "When do you want me to come?"

What Barbara said was true. Over the years my daily contacts with scores and scores of infants and children with Down syndrome allowed me to accumulate a considerable fund of personal knowledge about this population. There were times when this information enabled me to solve baffling health and developmental problems which other professionals, lacking firsthand experience, seemed unable to recognize or diagnose.

This intimate knowledge, I believed, allowed me to see the child with Down syndrome, not as a aberration, but as a human being, with the same need for love and attention, the same need to learn, to play, to make friends and to succeed as any other child. Although individuals with Down syndrome belong to a homogeneous group with certain basic characteristics that are prototypical to these people, each person has, within the conformity of this syndrome, his own strengths and weakness, his own uniqueness in appearance and personality. It was important, I learned, to differentiate between what might be considered "normal" for children with Down syndrome, and what, allowing for individual differences, was not. Any deviancy in health or behavior, outside the established perimeters of Down syndrome, was a signal to seek a cause, other than the obvious fact that the child in question had been born with an extra chromosome.

STRENGTHS

Contrary to what one may believe, children with Down syndrome have many strengths. First, when appropriate materials and instructional methods are used, they are able to learn with surprising acuity. Generally, fine-motor and cognitive activities are readily mastered although specific skills such as shoe-tying, buttoning and cutting with scissors usually take longer to achieve. Nevertheless, the obvious enjoyment and satisfaction of these children as they work with puzzles, colors, shapes, letters and words are a delight to behold.

Infants and toddlers with Down syndrome are also exceedingly responsive to shaping procedures which greatly simplify the task of teaching new skills. The word "shaping" refers to the technique of giving physical assistance by guiding a part of the child's body, arm, leg, fingers or hand to make the desired response.

"Touch your head," says the teacher in the process of teaching body parts to a young preschooler, and then assuming that the child may not know what is required, the teacher takes his hand and touches it to his head, teaching him the correct response to her command. Thus shaping is a way of physically showing a youngster what he or she must do until learning occurs and the proper response is made independently.

Turn-taking between teacher and child or between classmates is another successful method of instruction. The advantage of this approach is that it helps the child to be more interactive, a necessary skill for social development.

In addition to the general receptiveness that children with Down syndrome appear to have toward learning new tasks, as long as these tasks are based upon what they have already learned to do, they display yet another very important strength. This strength is the ability to discriminate between shapes, pictures, numbers, letters and words with remarkable accuracy at an early age. In spite of common vision problems, nearsightedness and strabismus (cross-eyedness) it is possible to capitalize upon this ability to teach developmental tasks of shape and color recognition as well as reading and counting and other functional age appropriate skills.

Even as an infant the child with Down syndrome is a reponsive social being. Kenny, a three-month-old baby, who attended the Infant Learning Class, was born with a cleft palate. This additional problem occurs in about 0.5 percent of the population. As a result of this defect, Kenny was unable to nurse well, and was tiny and frail. Yet, despite his physical weakness, Kenny's dark brown eyes gleamed with friendliness. When his mother looked at him and talked to him, he tried to "talk" in return. He moved his lips (now surgically repaired for harelip) in imitation of her lips movements and looked at her intently, communicating with his shining eyes and soft cooing sounds.

Although verbal expressive language (speech) tends to develop slowly among some children with Down syndrome, and in some cases poor articulation is difficult to overcome, receptive language is recognized as one of their strengths. Like many other positive characteristics of this population, this ability was not taken into consideration in the past. As we seek to maximize the potential of these strengths, it is important to remember that all children need and crave adult attention. Parents and teachers are the most significant persons in the life of a young child. If appropriate or desired behaviors are ignored, the child will instinctively find other, perhaps less desirable, ways of gaining the attention he wants. Teaching and childrearing methods that focus on positive feedback and praise when the child behaves or completes a task correctly is the best way of helping all children attain their fullest potential.

WEAKNESSES

Despite their many strengths and the higher expectations that we now have for children with Down syndrome, it would be unrealistic to deny the existence of a number of cognitive, physical and health problems. The majority are moderately or mildly mentally retarded. Severe mental retardation is rare, and if it exists it is usually the result of extreme environmental deprivation, brain damage, not generally associated with the syndrome, or it may even be caused by the presence of additional chromosomal abnormality not inherent to Down syndrome. Undiagnosed and untreated problems relating to hearing, the thyroid or seizures can also seriously delay development.

Hypotonia, poor muscle tone (flabbiness), small stature and flattened facial features are the major physical symptoms of this chromosomal difference. By age twelve the child with Down syndrome may be ten inches shorter than the average height for his age group. Growth hormones for these children is, in fact, a current medical issue.

In coloring, body height and build, however, children with Down syndrome like all children, tend to resemble their parents. It can be expected that children born to tall, slender parents will be taller and perhaps thinner than those born to shorter, heavier couples.

To a certain degree, intellectual development is also related to inherent parental intelligence, perhaps as a result of genetic as well as environmental factors.

Health may range from relatively good health to frequent upper respiratory infections, chronic otitis media (middle ear infection), congenital heart defects and other organic problems. Degrees of congenital heart defects are found in about 30 to 60 percent of the babies who are born with Down syndrome. These defects may range from a slight heart murmur to more serious cardiac malformations. The outlook for children with heart defects is much more sanguine now than it was in the past. Not only has open-heart surgery been perfected to the point where it is no longer considered a last-measure recourse, but the doctors themselves, no longer viewing these children as hopeless cases, unworthy of treatment, are more willing to intervene surgically and to repair the damage before it becomes life threatening. A number of people are now advocating routine echocardiograms for children with Down syndrome. A recent case in California where a woman with this syndrome received a heart and lung transplant illustrates the changing attitude on the part of the medical profession.

Another less-frequent congenital malformation results in an obstruction in the upper portion of the small intestine: duodenal stenosis or atresia. This problem must be remedied surgically as soon as it is discovered. Usually the problem is diagnosed shortly after birth. In some cases, however, it doesn't become apparent until the baby is several months old. Failure to gain weight and persistent regurgitation of food after eating should be viewed with suspicion.

In view of the number and the variability of the factors that may affect the behavior and health of the child with Down syndrome, it is easy to understand how a doctor, inexperienced in treating these children, may dismiss an inexplicable ailment as yet another manifestation of the syndrome, requiring no further investigation. This is what happened to Robin, and Lori, and a number of other children in my experience.

ROBIN*

Fran* and her newly adopted seven-month-old Down syndrome baby were waiting for me when I arrived on a scheduled visit to PRIDE, a preschool for disabled youngsters and one of our replication sites in Vancouver, Washington. The little girl, Robin, was a beautiful child with wavy black hair and large, lapis lazuli eyes, but she was exceedingly thin and pale, almost translucently white. Dark circles under her eyes accentuated her pallor and gave her the appearance of a famine-stricken waif.

I had met Fran before. We greeted each other warmly and she asked me to examine Robin, telling me how worried she was about her health and development. As I began my assessment I could see that although Robin appeared to be bright and alert, her muscle tone was poor, that she tired easily, and again I was struck by her thinness.

"How long have you had Robin?" I asked as I checked off an item on my assessment sheet.

"Four weeks, tomorrow ... "

"Has she gained any weight?"

"Not much, maybe an ounce or two. I don't see how she could, she spits up everything I give her."

At the end of my assessment, Fran brought out a baby bottle. Robin grasped it eagerly and hungrily gulped down the contents, but within minutes the food was regurgitated, spewing out in a fountain of curdled liquid. I tensed with alarm. Something was definitely wrong, and I believed I knew what it was.

"Has she been seen by a doctor?" I asked as we mopped up the mess.

"Oh, yes," the mother replied. "Our pediatrician claims it's nothing serious, that Robin will get over it, eventually."

I shook my head. "You should get another opinion. Take her to the University of Oregon Medical Center."

Nancy Warren*, PRIDE head teacher and coordinator, who had been sitting near by, rose to her feet. "I'll telephone and make an appointment."

"Yes, please do," Fran looked at her with troubled eyes. "I'm sick with worry."

Vancouver, Washington is situated on the north side of the magnificent Columbia river that flows between Washington and Oregon states. Portland, Vancouver's sister city, lies across the river. Washingtonians and Oregonians commute freely between the two cities, travelling back and forth across the Columbia River bridge. It would not be difficult for Fran to take her baby to the hospital.

An appointment was made for that afternoon. Fran telephoned me that night. My suspicions proved to be correct. A partial duodenal obstruction was diagnosed, and surgery was scheduled for the following morning. There was no time to lose. Robin was already so dehydrated and undernourished that a few more days' delay would have been fatal.

Robin and her family lived in a small farming community, an hour's drive from Vancouver. It is quite possible that her doctor had never treated an infant with Down syndrome before, and so didn't trouble to look beyond his stereotyped notion of what such a child might be like. Once again I found it necessary to urge parents not to accept glib answers in response to their concerns about their children's health and well being.

LITTLE STEVIE

"I'm concerned about little Steve," Nancy told me when I revisited the PRIDE program the following spring. "He's regressing."

I remembered Stevie, a smiling, docile little boy who entered the program at ten months of age about a year ago. I remembered his parents as well. A young couple, still in their teens, gentle, loving people, who adored Stevie. His mother, Heidi, had a sweet, round face, forget-me-not blue eyes, and curly hair, the color of freshly varnished pine. Stevie looked like his mother. He had the same sweet face, intensely blue eyes and fluffy hair. The whole family exuded such an appealing vulnerability that I was drawn to them with sincere affection.

"Oh," I said in response to Nancy's words. "I can hardly believe this. He was doing so well."

"Yes," she agreed. "He was. We were all encouraged by his progress."

When Stevie entered the program he did indeed show considerable delay in his physical development. I recalled, for example, how difficult it was for Stevie to pull himself up to a sitting position for he lacked the necessary strength in his arms and back to perform the exercise. Once he began attending the infant class and receiving physical therapy, however, he improved rapidly. Four months ago, when I last saw him, Stevie was sitting independently and using his arms and legs to push himself upright. Soon, we predicted, Stevie would begin walking around furniture.

"It's like it was in the beginning." Nancy went on, "He's not sitting without support any more, in fact he can hardly ... well, you better see for yourself," she concluded, leading the way into the classroom.

Stevie was on the floor, lying on a mat. I knelt down beside him.

"Hi, Stevie."

He turned his head slowly, met my eyes, but didn't smile. He looked tired.

"Come, sweetie, let's sit up."

I took his hands and gave a gentle tug. Instead of tensing his muscles and pulling himself forward to rise off the mat, Stevie allowed his head to drop backwards. It lolled like that of a newborn, his arms were limp in my grasp.

I had never encountered such a dramatic regression. Could it be his heart? I wondered. His record showed no congenital heart defects, but incipient problems are not always detected right away. Then I noticed something else, a yellowish tinge colored Stevie's face. Lifting his shirt I saw that his whole body appeared to have been dipped in a weak solution of iodine.

I glanced at Heidi who sat on the floor beside me, hands clenched on jean-clad knees.

"Does his skin look yellow to you?" I asked.

The young woman nodded. "I asked our doctor about it. He said it might be the diet. Told me not to feed Stevie carrots for awhile."

I didn't want to alarm her, but the color of his skin and his weakness troubled me.

"It may be more serious than that," I countered, trying to keep my voice noncommittal, but Heidi must have read something in my face. Her lip quivered.

"Something bad?" she whispered.

I met her eyes. "I don't know. But I think you should find out. Take him to the University of Oregon Medical Center," I recommended once again.

Stevie's parents followed my advice, and we received the fateful verdict. My fears were confirmed. Stevie had leukemia. Unfortunately a diagnosis doesn't always lead to a cure, and there was no hope for recovery. Within three weeks Stevie developed pneumonia and died.

LORI

Barbara Thomas and I finalized our plans for the workshop and I flew to Macon the following month. I arrived on a Friday evening and checked in at a gracious old hotel where a room had been reserved for me. The next morning Barbara came to the hotel to drive me to a nearby auditorium for my presentation. After corresponding for almost two years, this was the first time that we met face to face. I was surprised by her appearance. At thirty-eight she looked old and dowdy. Although it was the middle of March and the weather was pleasantly warm, Barbara was wearing a heavy, garishly green wool coat. The coat looked expensive but the color was exceedingly unbecoming and the coat itself was too long and bulky for her small frame. I had the impression that the coat had been bought, and was now worn, blindly — something to pull off a rack and out of a closet, uncaring about its appearance or the weather.

Above the odious green her face looked drawn and sallow. A perpetual frown carved severe lines across her forehead. Parenthetical grooves, from nose to chin, bracketed a bitter mouth.

"I'm so glad you came!" Barbara clasped my hand smiling, briefly lifting the sagging corners of her sorrowful mouth. But the warmth of her greeting failed to lighten the bleakness in her large amber-flecked hazel eyes.

Barbara could be pretty, I thought. Her features were attractive. Her short, reddish brown hair matched her lashes and brows, and the amber highlights in her eyes.

It was humid in the car. Barbara removed her coat and threw it on the back seat. She was dressed in a faded cotton blouse, an old gray skirt.

Putting her Mercedes Benz in gear, Barbara sighed as if reading my thoughts.

"I should get some new clothes, but I don't have the energy to shop." The lines on her face became more pronounced, "I'm just too tired to care."

I nodded in sympathy. "Lori has so many needs. It's been hard for you."

"Terribly hard. I feel as if I'm running down endless corridors, seeking a way out, but all the doors are locked or lead only to a dead end. Sometimes I simply want to fall asleep — or disappear — and pretend that none of this ever happened ... If only ... if only ... " She broke off and forced herself into a brighter mood.

"That's why I'm glad you're here. I'm sure you'll be able to help Lori."

"I hope I can." I answered softly, acutely aware of her pain, the crushing depression that gripped her and which the carelessness of her dress, the tight, creased face, the lifeless eyes revealed.

Only another parent coping with the ceaseless demands of an ailing, disabled infant could understand Barbara's depression, the debilitating frustration of her search as she turned from one physician to another, seeking relief for her suffering child. I had counseled and tried to help many such parents, often feeling that doctors, who could be kind and supportive towards parents of normal sick children, were frequently surprisingly indifferent to the desperate need of fathers and mothers whose young were sick as well as disabled.

When we arrived the auditorium was filled to capacity with parents of children with disabilities, special education teachers and other professionals. Armed with slides, video tapes, overhead transparencies and handouts, I launched into my topic. I spoke on typical child development, how it compared to that of children with special needs and on strategies for maximizing the potential of that population. It was a full day workshop, but I had an attentive audience and the hours passed quickly. At four-thirty as I was fielding the final questions from the participants, I caught Barbara's eye. Her frown had deepened. We were running overtime and she was anxious for us to adjourn, anxious to take me home with her to meet Lori. I had hoped to meet Frank, Barbara's husband, as well, but he was away on a business trip.

The Thomases and their children, two teenaged sons and Lori lived in a stately brick house on a tree-lined street. A lush green lawn, rosebushes and other shrubs surrounded the house. A peach tree was budding into bloom at the back.

"Please sit down. I'll get Lori." Barbara ushered me into a formal living room as if I were an oracle entering a temple. I stepped across a thick, jewel-toned oriental rug and selected an arm chair upholstered in gray velvet. Lace curtains hung over the windows. A mirror in an ornate gilt frame and several fine oils decorated the walls. White roses, arranged in a crystal bowl, stood on a highly polished mahogany table. It was a beautiful room reflecting elegance and money. I looked about the room, remembering Polly, the squalid shabbiness of the Stokes home. Once again it occurred to me that children with Down syndrome and other disabling conditions happen among all the races, at all levels of society, rich, or poor, no one is immune.

Barbara returned carrying Lori. They were followed by a young black woman, Lori's nanny. Seemingly, the child was dressed for a party. Ruffles and lace trimmed her frilly pink frock. A small pink bow adorned a strand of wispy blond hair. Obviously Barbara's present indifference to her own appearance didn't apply to Lori's.

"Here she is!" There was love and pride in Barbara's voice.

I rose and took Lori into my arms. She felt as light and fragile as an empty egg shell. She was not an attractive child. Her finery couldn't conceal the thin, undersized body, the boney ridges of her spine, her spindly limbs, nor the lankness of her hair, so lovingly brushed and curled for my visit. She didn't look like a child, her tiny face was a shrivelled, miniature version of an old woman's face, features furrowed by suffering.

Nanny Martha May spread a blanket on the floor. I laid Lori upon it and knelt beside her. Lori began to whine, a tearless, complaining moan.

"Oh, she's crying again!" Martha May clasped her hands hopelessly. "Why does she do it so much!"

"I don't know." I began stroking Lori's stomach, something I did to soothe fretful babies. The moaning stopped.

Barbara joined me on the blanket. "'Let her sit," she urged. "See if she'll sit for you."

I took hold of Lori's hands and gave a gentle tug. Contrary to what I expected, her muscles tightened, her match-stick fingers clutched mine as she pulled herself, quickly and adroitly, to a sitting position. There was a wiry strength in that skinny little frame, I discovered.

"She has good muscle tone," I told Barbara. "Look how well she's holding her head." Lori was sitting with absolute poise, her back ramrod straight, her legs lightly flexed, and crossed at the ankles. I slipped a bracelet off my arm and held it out to Lori. A flicker of pleasure lightened her wasted little face as she reached for it, extending her right arm with perfect ease and without losing her balance. For a few seconds she held the bracelet, examining it, turning it in her hands, then, without warning, she toppled backwards, forcibly, as if someone had given her a sharp nudge. For an instant Lori lay where she had fallen, unmoving, then she resumed her eerie wail. Once again I rubbed her tummy, and once again she stopped.

Barbara grasped my arm, her eyes, peering anxiously into mine.

"You saw what happened! You saw how she fell. It happens all the time, no matter how much we try to make her sit."

"We'll try it again," I told Barbara.

Brought to an upright position, Lori sat as before, looking comfortable and pleased with herself. Then, after a minute or two, she again lost control and tumbled to the floor. This time, however, I watched Lori closely. The instant before she fell, I noted something that I had been half expecting to see — a fleeting blankness in her expression, a sudden stare, a cessation of movement in her eyes.

"What is it? Did you see something? Do you know what's wrong?" Barbara persisted, suddenly aware of my watchfulness.

"Not yet, but I think ... I think I have a clue."

The third time Lori toppled over, I was convinced that we were witnessing an akinetic convulsion. Different from the severe grand mal seizures that anyone can recognize, the akinetic, the petit mal and some other forms of epileptic seizures are much more elusive. As brief as the flicker of a malfunctioning light, these attacks are of such short duration that they can be difficult to pinpoint. A petit mal seizure, for example, can appear as a sudden, momentary blank stare, or a rapid blinking of eyes accompanied, sometimes, by small twitching movements. An akinetic convulsion is manifested by sudden, transient muscular collapse, such as Lore exhibited. However fleeting these repetitive episodes of unconsciousness may be, the fact that they may recur almost continuously, from five to two hundred times a day, makes them sufficiently disruptive as to seriously interfere with normal learning and development. Any suspected seizure activity should therefore be properly diagnosed and controlled with drugs.

I turned to Barbara. "Has Lori been seen by a neurologist?"

"No, why?" Her tone was suddenly sharp with apprehension.

"I can't be sure, of course, but I suspect that the reason Lori can neither sit nor stand is because she's having akinetic seizures."

The mother blanched and her voice sank to a whisper.

"Epilepsy?"

"Oh, Lord!" Martha May clapped her hands to her mouth, her eyes wide with horror.

"It's not so bad," I began, but Barbara wasn't listening. Springing to her feet she whirled upon me in a flash of hysterical anger.

"How dare you! How dare you say such a thing! What do you know? You're not a pediatrician! Lori has been seen by all kinds of medical doctors. No one, not one, ever mentioned epilepsy!" She turned and walked away from me, tears rolling down the grooves in her cheeks.

Dismayed, I chided myself. I should have been more circumspect. I should have remembered the fragile vulnerability of parents whose children are disabled, I should have remembered too, that old myths and superstitions are hard to overcome. Epilepsy is still a "dangerous" word.

Derived from the Greek word for seizures, epilepsy has been known to mankind for a long time. Hippocrates describes the disorder in his *Work*, and there is a reference to it in the *New Testament*. Through the ages, however, because the sudden twitchings, convulsions and lapses into unconsciousness of the "falling sickness" were so difficult to understand, epilepsy remained a mysterious ailment, misunderstood and misrepresented through folklore and superstition. It is now known that epileptic seizures are caused by an abnormal and recurrent discharge of excessive nervous energy within the brain. It is also recognized that the outward manifestations of the disorder, the convulsions, the twitchings, unconsciousness and mental disturbances indicate underlying dysfunction within the brain or central nervous system.

In some instances the causes precipitating seizure activity can be readily determined. In other instances they are more obscure and unidentifiable. No one symptom is an essential feature of the disease. Generally, however, brain damage as a result of an accident, congenital defect or birth injury, pathological changes in the brain developing after an infection such as meningitis or encephalitis; cerebral abscess and tumors, as well as heredity are among the main causes of epilepsy. In Lori's case, I suspected that her seizures resulted from a defect in her nervous system or a birth injury.

Despite this knowledge, and despite the fact that few people believe in witchcraft and demons, the reality of epilepsy still evokes strong reactions of fear, and persons suffering from this disorder are still discriminated against, shunned and rejected.

I remember an incident that occurred on a city bus that I was riding many years ago. I was eighteen at the time, a junior in college. As the bus weaved its way through Seattle downtown traffic, a woman, seated across the aisle from me, suffered a grand mal seizure. There was immediate pandemonium. Someone screamed.

Disregarding traffic, the driver jerked the vehicle to a stop, flung the door open and leaped from the bus. A few passengers followed his example, fleeing as from a holocaust. Meanwhile the poor woman was convulsing, thrashing about, slamming her head against the metal bar across the back of her seat. I glanced around the bus. The remaining passengers sat in frozen immobility, gaping with wide eyes. Would no one come to her aid? Thinking of the injuries the woman might sustain from the repeated banging, I rose from my place and cupped my hands under her jerking head, cushioning the blows. Her hair felt soft and springy against my palms. I stood at my post, listening to the crescendoing siren of an approaching ambulance. A few minutes later the driver returned followed by a policeman and ambulance attendants. The woman, who by now had fallen into a deep sleep, was laid on a stretcher and carried away.

I acted instinctively, seeking neither praise nor recognition, but I was surprised when I resumed my seat that no one spoke to me, no one commented on what had happened. I felt, in fact, a drawing away, a shunning, as if I had somehow become contaminated, as if I too had become in their view a "freak."

Although this was my first encounter with a grand mal seizure in a person, I had been neither frightened nor repelled. Once, as a child, I saw my grandmother administering to a puppy who was having repeated convulsions, and who was destined to die of his illness. In those days there was no vaccine against distemper, that dreaded canine disease.

Lori, still on the blanket where she had fallen, began to whine again, her little old woman's face contorting as if with pain. I lifted Lori and placed her on my lap. Martha May nodded towards the child.

"Is it ... is it all right to pick her up?"

I looked at her questioningly.

"Won't ... won't it make her have ... another ... fit?"

"I don't think you'd notice if she did. No," I added, "it won't hurt her. Lori isn't changed by what happened. She's no different from what she was five minutes ago. Very likely she's been having seizures from the day she was born, only no one ever noticed them before."

I then explained that as long as Lori was neither sitting nor standing the muscular collapse of an akinetic episode would not be apparent.

Recovering from her tantrum, Barbara sank on the rug beside me and wiped her eyes with a crumpled tissue.

"I'm sorry I spoke to you the way I did. It was very rude of me. I'm sure you're right."

"I didn't mean to frighten you."

Lori turned to her mother and held out her arms. Smiling sorrowfully Barbara cuddled her little girl, stroking the limp, yellow hair.

"Poor baby, poor little Lori. Already she's suffered so much ... and now ... now you tell me something else is wrong ... will she ever get well?" A fresh tear glistened on the golden-brown lashes. "Lori's very precious to me, you know that, don't you?"

"Yes, I do, and I know how distressing this is for you, but you mustn't despair. Seizure disorders are fairly common," I continued, trying to reassure her, "proper diagnosis and medication can bring them under control."

"Is this why Lori cries so much, because she has seizures?"

"Perhaps, indirectly. Lori appears to be in pain. It may be a stomach inflammation," I replied, avoiding the words gastritis and ulcer which came to mind. "Epilepsy is an extremely unpredictable disease. It has been known to cause a variety of abdominal upsets, so we mustn't dismiss that possibility," I concluded.

No longer belligerent, Barbara nodded in agreement. "Something is definitely wrong. Lori is so thin. I'm worried sick about her poor appetite, her slow weight gain."

I glanced at my wristwatch. It was time to leave for the airport.

"May I phone for a cab?" I asked.

"Oh, no, I'll drive you," Barbara protested, handing Lori to Martha May.

On the way to the airport Barbara again apologized for her outburst and thanked me repeatedly for seeing Lori and for my advice. As she spoke Barbara became visibly more relaxed, the harsh lines on her face softened, becoming less disfiguring. I judged that her angry eruption, prompted by her fear, frustration, despair, and perhaps never fully expressed until that moment, served to lighten the depression that enveloped her.

About a month later I received an ecstatic letter from Barbara. A neurological examination confirmed my suspicions. Lori was indeed having akinetic seizures. Once adjusted doses of phenobarbitol brought the disorder under control, Lori no longer toppled over, and was now able to sit for indefinite periods of time. She was also learning to crawl and stand. Furthermore, X-rays revealed that Lori had an ulcer. Although the exact cause of this problem was not determined it also responded to treatment. Lori's appetite improved, the continual whining stopped, and she had actually gained two and a half pounds.

A year later I returned to give a second workshop in Macon. This time I saw Lori at the developmental center where she was now attending a preschool toddler class on a daily basis. Lori was sitting in a high chair when I arrived, eating a peanut butter sandwich with gusto. Although still small for her age, the pathetic little face had filled out; healthy flesh rounded her bones, and even the limp hair had developed a salubrious sheen and thickness. Lori still had a great deal of catching up to do in her cognitive and physical skills, and she was still highly susceptible to colds and infections, but on the whole she had become a healthier, happier child. Barbara, too, had lost her haggard, worried look. No longer despairing, her bright smile made her young and attractive. After this last visit, Barbara's letters ceased to arrive. I took that to mean that all was well, that Lori was continuing to make progress and that Barbara could lay some of her earlier, tormenting concerns aside.

It was fortunate, in a way, that Lori's akinetic seizures were confirmed so readily. This is not always the case, and as it sometimes happens brain scans fail to reveal any abnormality, making it difficult, even impossible, for a parent or teacher to convince a neurologist that a child is indeed having seizures. Such was the case with Shawna.

SHAWNA

Shawna was a child with Down syndrome attending the toddler class at the Experimental Education Unit. She was a well coordinated, outgoing youngster who promised to be a star pupil. Penny, our loving, fiercely dedicated teacher whose battle on behalf of little Maggie was described in the first chapter of this book, was delighted with Shawna's progress.

"Shawna's so bright," Penny boasted to me. "She must have a near normal I.Q. Do you know that in one week she learned to read her name and ten other words, all the labels that I have around the classroom: table, chair, window, piano ... ?"

"Wonderful!" I agreed.

A few days later I met Penny in the hall. She looked unhappy. "What's wrong?" I asked.

Penny gave me a sullen look, "Everything!"

"How come?"

"Oh, Shawna screwed up my data."

The teachers, I knew, kept a daily record of the pupils' progress. After three days of consistently correct performance a child was moved on to the next step in his program. I assumed that Shawna had failed to meet this goal.

"Didn't she reach criterion?"

"She didn't even try!"

"Perhaps she was bored, or you've been pushing her too hard."

Penny squared her slight shoulders indignantly. "I know when a child is bored, and I know better than to push a child!" she declared, offended by my words.

I smiled, apologizing. "What do you think happened?"

"I don't know. She was just ... spacey ... like she wasn't even there. The same thing happened at juice time and music. I had to call her name three times before she took notice and reached for a cracker."

"What happened at music time?"

"Same thing. She took the rhythm sticks and then just sat, holding them, staring into space."

"You checked her hearing?"

"Of course. I took her to next door to CDMRC for an evaluation right after class."

"And?"

"Normal, for both ears."

Ear infections with the accompanying accumulation of fluid in the inner ear and the resulting hearing impairment is one of the most significant problems among young children with Down syndrome, so it was not surprising that both Penny and I immediately thought to check Shawna's hearing before seeking other reasons for her strange behavior.

Many children with Down syndrome who had been referred to me by parents or teachers seeking advice on the child's lack of attention, delayed language development or hyperactive, disruptive behaviors, were found, after I had recommended a hearing evaluation by an audiologist, to be suffering from chronic ear infections. It is important that these evaluations be done by a specialist because the ear canals of children with Down syndrome are so small and irregular that it is often impossible for a doctor to detect any abnormality during a routine office examination of the ears.

In Shawna's case, however, we had to seek another cause. For a few days after my conversation with Penny, Shawna reverted to her previous responsive behavior. Then just as Penny began to think of the child's inattentiveness as a one time occurrence, it happened again. Penny began keeping track of these incidents. After several more episodes, Penny concluded that Shawna was having petit mal seizures. We decided it was time to discuss our suspicions with the little girl's parents.

It turned out that Shawna's parents had also noticed these periods of blanking out, but since their daughter's overall development and behavior was so exceptional, they dismissed these episodes as insignificant, fleeting moments of daydreaming. Nevertheless, when Penny suggested taking Shawna to a neurologist the parents agreed willingly, showing none of Lori's mother's emotional reaction.

By now I shared Penny's conviction that Shawna had a seizure disorder, and we were both greatly surprised when the results of her EEG (electroencephalogram) proved to be negative. Relieved, Shawna's parents accepted the verdict, but not Penny.

"I know Shawna's having petit mal seizures, but no one will believe me!" Penny complained. "I wish I could make that neurologist come here, and see for himself ... the trouble is, I can't predict when she's going to get spacey again."

About a week later Penny announced that she had a plan.

"I'm going to video tape Shawna. I'll borrow a camera from Media Services and get her seizures on tape!"

From then on Penny kept the camera at her side, and before long her vigilance was rewarded. Once again Shawna experienced several episodes in one day. The result was a convincing video tape which Penny triumphantly presented to Shawna's parents and the neurologist. The evidence was conclusive. Shawna was placed on medication and her attacks, temporal lobe seizures, became a thing of the past.

Once more Penny's vigilance and dedication served to help a child in need.

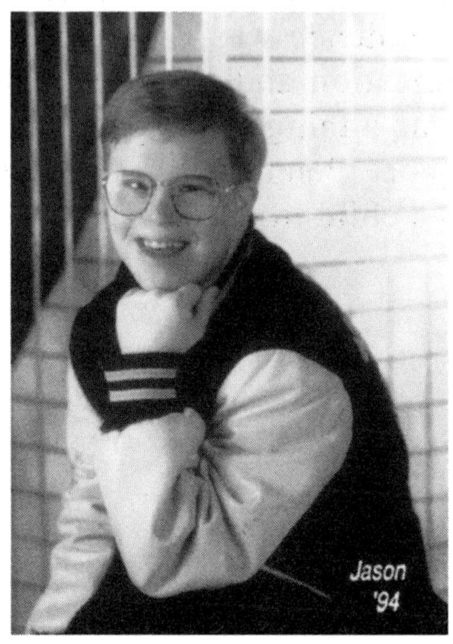

A graduation photo of Jason Marick, age 19, wearing the letterman's jacket he received for a job well done, as manager of his high school's basketball team.

Chapter Eleven
Tears and Triumphs

The overhead lamp cast a hard white light on the stainless steel, the chrome and the gleaming tiles of the delivery room. Lying on the table, her raised knees draped with a hospital-green sheet, Pamela Jones was oblivious to the light just as she was to the capped, masked, rubber-gloved, green-robed figures surrounding her. Focused on the primeval task of bringing forth a new life, her body had become a single-minded machine, laboring irrevocably towards that single resolution. Her breath came in short, practiced pants. Perspiration matted her hair and dripped down her face. Her fingers, clenching the hands of one of the shrouded figures, whitened with the strength of her gripping. Mounting waves of pain, relentless as an incoming tide, rolled over her; but she was prepared, and met each onslaught with augmenting effort.

"Once more," came the mask-muffled voice of the physician. "Push now, push harder, you're almost there."

Muscles strained to the utmost, a climax of pain, and then suddenly, incredible release as something solid yet resilient slid forth through her parted thighs. She heard the thin wail of her newborn's cry.

Exhausted, relief flooding her senses, Pamela sank back on the pillow. A wary stillness settled over the room.

"It's a boy," the doctor spoke at last in a cold, flat voice.

Unerringly Pamela caught that flatness, the ominous silence. Alarm jangled her nerves.

"What's wrong!" She struggled to sit up. If's something wrong with my baby!"

Someone patted her shoulder and eased her back to the pillow.

"Lie still, honey, everything will be all right."

"I want to see my baby!"

"Hush now, you need to rest."

Pamela felt the quick, cold swab of an alcohol drenched cotton, the sting of a needle. The room tilted and she slid into oblivion.

When Pamela awoke, she lay in a quiet, darkened room. A white coverlet stretched snugly across her legs. The steady throb of passing cars reached her ears like the distant boom of breaking surf. A late afternoon sun, finding cracks in the partially closed louvered blinds striped the ceiling with pale, yellow bars. *Where was she?* Trying to orient herself, her hand reached out to touch the familiar mound of her pregnant body. Her hand fell on a flat surface ... gone was the protruding roundness. Pamela jerked to full consciousness. It hadn't been a dream. It had really happened. Her baby had actually been born. As memory returned so did the sense of alarm, the foreboding that something was wrong. *Was the feeling real, or was it part of a dream?*

Pamela turned her head to reach for the call button. A man sat slumped in a chair, a hand covering his face. Robert! Joy quickened her heart beat. Robert, her husband, was here! Together they attended child birth classes, practiced her breathing and planned that he would be her coach during delivery, but when labor started, ten days ahead of time, Robert was at a construction site, seventy miles south of Seattle.

"Robert?"

He rose quickly and came to her side. As she circled his shoulders with her arms and lifted her face for his kiss, he dropped his head and began to sob.

Certainty hit her like a thunderbolt. Her baby was dead!

"Pamela?"

Dr. Ketterson spoke as he entered the room, carrying a small, blanket-swathed bundle. Robert walked to the window, and turning his back, surreptitiously wiped his eyes. The doctor's appearance, however, had banished her fears. Robert wept for joy, Pamela decided. She held out her arms and smiled.

"Is he all right?"

The doctor approached, but there was no answering smile. "Yes, he has all of his fingers and toes, and he's a healthy baby, if that's what you mean."

"Oh, I'm so glad. So happy! My baby, give him to me." She smiled radiantly, reaching for the bundle.

Ketterson looked at her, his eyes growing dark with compassion. "I'm very sorry, but I must tell you what I already told your husband. Your baby is basically healthy, but he has Down syndrome."

"What do you mean!" Her voice turned hoarse, ugly.

"Mongolism. Your baby is a mongoloid." The doctor attempted to lower the infant into her arms, but she flinched as if the blue blanket contained a coiled cobra. "No, it's not true! Not my baby, this is not my baby. I don't want it. Take it away!" She flung herself towards the wall and burst into tears.

The doctor shifted uneasily, cleared his throat. "We'll talk later." Quietly, almost furtively, he laid the blanket-wrapped infant across the bed, and just as quietly left the room, shutting the door behind him.

Once again Robert took her into his arms. Husband and wife, mother and father, clung to each other, mingling their tears, and all the while their infant son lay between them sleeping peacefully.

Finally, her tears subsiding, Pamela reached for a Kleenex, wiped her eyes and blew her nose.

"Oh, Robert, what are we going to do?"

Robert raised his head and looked into her reddened eyes.

"What do you think we should do?"

"He's our baby."

"Yes."

"Do you ... do you ... " her voice dropped to a whisper, "know anything about ... about ... mongolism."

"Down syndrome? Only what the doctor told me. We'll have to learn won't we?"

"Yes."

The baby snuffled in his sleep and gave a little hiccup.

Pamela tensed with apprehension. "Have you seen him, does ... does he look ... very awful?"

"I don't know ... shall we look?"

Robert reached for the bundled baby, and laid him by her side. Holding her breath, Pamela drew back the blanket with trembling fingers.

Her breath came out with a swoosh, and her voice cracked in a little laugh.

"Robert, he's cute! Look at his hair, it's curly!"

"And red, just like yours."

"I had no idea ... I was so afraid ... but, he's adorable ... He's ... he's just like ... a baby."

She clasped the infant to her breast and dropped a kiss on his silky curls. Fresh tears glistened in her eyes, tears of relief and love. The first bonding between mother and child had begun.

"But he still has Down syndrome," Robert warned.

"I know."

"He will be slower to develop, the doctor told me. He will need special help and training ... "

Holding her baby with one arm, Pamela grasped her husband's hand with the other. "But we'll do it, won't we? We'll give him all the help he needs ... and ... and we'll love him, and care for him and accept him, no matter how much or how little he can do."

Robert squeezed her hand in return, "Of course, he's our son, and I love you both, very, very much."

Robert and Pamela may not be actual people, yet they are real in the sense that their experience as I described it, is based upon the true experiences of couples that I have known. For every couple that is overcome by the trauma of a disabled child, there are many others who are able to make a successful transition from initial grieving to acceptance, love and positive activity.

As I think of the couples that inspired me to write about Pamela and Robert, I remember Judy and James Marick* and their son, Jason*. The Maricks live in Vancouver, Washington, and I met them and Jason, a lively infant, with a cap of glossy reddish blond hair, in my hotel room where I was staying during a conference at which I was one of the speakers.

Prior to our meeting Judy had written to me, seeking help with Jason, because there were no early intervention programs in the area. Recognizing their need and the need of other families in the same circumstances, and after talking to Judy in person, I offered to help her establish an infant and preschool program in her community.

The enterprise was highly successful and in a short time evolved, under the auspices of the Clark Community College, into the PRIDE program. With Judy's unfailing dedication and under Nancy Warren's expertise as teacher and coordinator the program flourished and continues to do so. In 1985 PRIDE celebrated the tenth anniversary of its existence. From the day of its inception until he entered public school at age six, Jason participated in the program. Jason is now a high school graduate, a young man with a keen interest in the theater and acting, having performed in a number of local productions.

Over the years I've had many opportunities to speak with parents of newborn babies, toddlers and preschoolers, but since my focus has always been on the early years, I've had less contact with parents of older children, and less opportunity to learn from them about their particular difficulties, their fears, frustrations as well as their joys and hopes as the children that I knew as preschoolers matured into young adulthood. In hopes of bridging this gap in my experience, I asked Judy Marick to share with me her thoughts and feelings as the mother of a maturing son with special needs. This is what she wrote.

"For twenty-one years, as Jason's mother, adjustment to all the barriers of fear, prejudice, lack of understanding, preconceived expectations, stereotypical attitudes of others and society in general has been my greatest difficulty. These barriers are the most difficult to eliminate, and the most difficult for me, as a parent, to understand. I'm often frustrated by the seemingly daily need to "teach": it's okay to be different, to learn in a different way or at a slower speed, to speak or hear or love in a different way. We can't all be alike.

Jason is a boy with all the emotions, feelings, potential of any boy; he is a boy with all the dreams and hopes of a job, girl friend, apartment, marriage, and travel.

"It has been and is very draining of my emotional and time resources to continually work with the educational system to place Jason in classes where demands are made of him, to give Jason opportunities to risk and as a result be challenged to a higher level. I've always found that given the opportunity, he is increasingly able to prove that he is more alike than different. Through the mainstreamed experiences, the "differences" become familiar and don't seem so important. Jason is differently able. I have found that if I treat Jason as I expect him to be, he will be all that he can be.

"I must say, though, that with all the extra concerns, work, and worry financially, medically, and educationally, I would not want Jason any different. The challenges and rewards of having Jason as one of our six children has given our family a bonding and an awareness of the goodness of life. He has such an appreciation and awareness of this great God-given world. His gentleness, love, caring, politeness and infectious laughter makes us all smile in a relaxed manner of acceptance of each other and our own capabilities whatever they are.

"Also I must recognize the fact, that because of Jason, we have met and made some of the most wonderful lifelong friends. They are my support system, my emotional and often spiritual strength providers.

"It is deeply satisfying to know that because of Jason, many of the professional and educational people have new and higher expectations of all people, have less fear, ignorance and prejudice, that some of the barriers are being eliminated, and more dreams are becoming realities."

Judy concluded her letter with this postscript: "Monday, Jason and Michael Pendergraft* (a friend and classmate with Down syndrome) are to be tested to receive their first belt in Karate. The boys have been taking classes since last October. They love it, and their teacher is wonderful. Our local paper is covering the event.

"On Wednesday, I'm speaking to the students and faculty at Jason's school about what it is like to parent a child who is handicapped. Should be interesting."

The tears that are shed upon the birth of a child with special needs are real, the bewilderment, the heartaches and grieving are genuine, but the human spirit is resilient and in most cases parents are able to meet the challenge with courage and determination. Parents like Judy and James Marick and others who battle against the barriers Judy describes; parents who agitate for quality education and who persevere in the face of all difficulties to assure social, educational and vocational opportunities for their children are the victors. As a result of their unflagging efforts, fathers and mothers have the joy of seeing their children, once believed to be incapable of achieving even the most rudimentary life skills, realize heretofore undetected and unfulfilled potentials. These parents have the joy of seeing their children function as self-sufficient individuals, intellectually, socially, and economically — this is their reward and triumph.

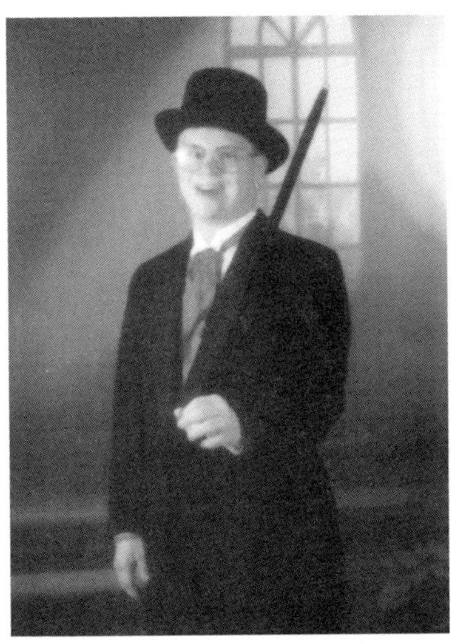

Jason Marick in the role of Freddie Eynsford-Hill from My Fair Lady.

Chapter Twelve
The Poet from Yemen and The Plight of Fathers

If I had the power, son,
I would build your bones
and impart intellect in your brain.
I would spend my life
so you may live unhandicapped and
I sleep comfortably,
because you won't starve or die of thirst. Fear haunts
me, that you may suffer, after my death,
in a world, where generosity is complete meanness.
I wish you knew how much I think of you,
how ill I be, when you are sick; how sleepless I remain
and how much I pity those in agony, because you teach
me goodness and love and how innocence is a bliss.
Had I been told that your good health lies
in the oceans' depths
I would have plunged into those raging waves; or if it
were on the highest peaks,
I would have climbed the mysterious heights, or were
it be in the far stars,

I would have flown with death-challenging wings.
But alas my son, we live in the East, where human lives are valueless and man in turn could not care less.

This poem was written and translated from Arabic by the man I call The Poet from Yemen, Ali Mahammad Luqman*, the father of a fourteen-year-old boy with Down syndrome. I believe this poem is a fitting introduction to what I want to say about fathers. Although the preceding chapter was devoted to the emotional impact of having a handicapped child and how it can affect the lives of the people involved, such a discussion would not be complete without a special word about the particular plight of fathers. Society doesn't always recognize that fathers hurt too, and that the birth of a baby with Down syndrome or some other defect can affect them as deeply as it does the mother. True, the mother is generally the one to bear the immediate burden of care and she does not always have the outlets offered by a job or career, especially during the crucial first few months of the new baby's life. On the other hand, the mother can become involved in an infant learning program where she can meet other women with whom she can share problems and concerns. She can also, when pressures become too great, find relief in tears without social censure.

Fathers, however, are expected to go on about their business of earning a living with little thought by anyone of the emotional pain they may be suffering. Men are generally not permitted to weep in public or private, nor are they able to talk freely about self-doubts, or feelings of helplessness, frustration, shame, or any emotion that might imply weakness or lack of masculinity. Also, the opportunity of meeting and talking with fathers of other handicapped children is not readily available. Nevertheless, the problems and the hurt are real.

The sad case of a friend who shot himself illustrates the extremity of the conflicts that a father may experience. Few men in his situation commit suicide, however, the disproportionate number of divorced men among fathers of Down syndrome children suggests an abnormally high incidence of unresolved distress.

Once, while addressing a large group of parents in Tokyo, I spoke on this topic. After my words had been translated by an interpreter, a man rose from his chair, tears streaming down his face. His infant son was born with Down syndrome, he told me, speaking in English; this was the first time that anyone acknowledged the pain in his heart, and this was the first time he felt able to share his grief. Repeating his testimony in Japanese, the man sat down to a burst of sympathetic applause, while many other men and women wept openly. So much for Asian stoicism, I thought, welcoming their tears as a healing process.

Programs that provide early intervention to infants and their mothers should also provide a special time for fathers. Such a program, initiated as part of the infant learning program at the University of Washington, proved highly successful. Fathers and their children came to a Saturday morning class twice a month.

The program[9] focused on father-child interaction. Fathers were taught how to relate to their baby through songs, games, and basic gross-motor exercises. In addition to the father-child aspects of the program, the men had an opportunity to listen to a male speaker, usually a pediatrician, dentist, educator, or lawyer, speak on a topic of general interest. The morning ended with refreshments for babies and adults, and an informal discussion.

It was significant, I thought, that men with younger babies looked for advice from fathers of older children in the same way that the mothers sought help and counsel from each other. Another positive spin-off from these sessions was the increased sharing between husband and wife, and general total family involvement in their baby's development.

THE POET FROM YEMEN

I met Mr. Ali Luqman in 1978 on a Friday afternoon in late October when he came to the University to see me. He was accompanied by Gala*, his son, Gala's older brother, a doctor in the American Army, who, I noticed in passing, was carrying a musical instrument in a case, and three women. Mr. Luqman and his sons wore western clothing, dark suits, white shirts and ties, but the women were shrouded in flowing black robes. Although the women were not veiled, their dark, remote faces were lost in the shadows of their draperies.

Of medium height and build, with silvered black hair and light copper-toned skin, Luqman was an attractive man, and I felt drawn to him, to the gentleness in his face and to the compelling intensity in his dark eyes — eyes that glowed with the light of a deep, inner flame.

Luqman greeted me graciously and introduced his companions. One of the women was his wife, the other two were her sisters. After shaking hands with the men I turned to the women, but they stood apart, huddled together, silent and motionless like statues. Speaking flawless English, in a cultured voice, Luqman explained that after he, his wife and sisters-in-law returned to Yemen, Gala would remain with his brother in order to attend school in America. This was why he was asking me to assess Gala and to recommend an appropriate school program for the boy.

It was after working hours and the building was deserted. As I led my party down empty halls to a classroom where I had prepared materials for my evaluation, the only sound was the distant burr of a floor polisher the custodian was using in another area.

I placed myself across a small table from Gala. Acting as our interpreter, Mr. Luqman sat on my right. The rest of the family took chairs a few feet away. Our session began with a general assessment of Gala's intellectual ability. Because of the language barrier I chose the Peabody Picture Vocabulary Test. This is a nonverbal assessment that can be administered to children of all ages as well as to adults. The test itself is composed of a series of pictures, ranging from simple, familiar objects to the portrayal of increasingly complex abstract ideas and a correspondingly more difficult vocabulary. Each page of the Peabody contains four pictures representing objects, animals, actions or ideas. The student is required to point to what he believes is the correct response when the examiner names one of the four illustrations on each page. The test measures language comprehension as well as intellectual awareness and understanding of the environment.

Gala performed very well, scoring in the moderately to mildly mentally retarded range. He was a quiet, well-behaved boy, who worked with equal willingness and concentration on the additional academic tasks that I set before him. At the end of the evaluations, Dr. Luqman opened the instrument case that he had been carrying and handed Gala a guitar.

"May he play for you?" Mr. Luqman asked me.

"Of course!"

Strumming the guitar in accompaniment, Gala sang an Arabian folk song. It was a pleasing, harmonious performance. Although there were obvious gaps in Gala's education, and he had yet to learn English, I assured his family that he was indeed a capable young boy, who should be able to adjust to school and life in America, and I congratulated his parents on their efforts on his behalf. In a land where there is little tolerance of differences, Ali Luqman was a loving father. He accepted Gala, believed in his potential and taught him as much as he could.

A short time later I received the following letter from The Poet from Yemen and a copy of his poem.

Dear Mrs. Dmitriev,

As I am now on my way home, I wish to record my deep gratitude to you for the valuable time you have given my son, Gala, and the expert opinion you have very kindly given me about him. His mother, brother and I are indeed most thankful. We are deeply touched by your kindness to such boys and girls, your sympathy with their loving but helpless parents and your immense aid and assistance to create smiles on the faces of depressed fathers and mothers.

Your opinion has rectified much of the misconceptions we were led to believe about him. In our countries we do not yet have helpful experts like your goodself to resort to when confronted with such problems and no official or charitable organizations exist to take such retarded children into their warmth.

I have once written a long Arabic poem about mentally retarded children, which was published by the daily paper in my country. As a reaction, I got all the sympathies of the society in which other fathers with different sons' and daughters' problems shared my vexation and care. They advised that having a son to stay with in Washington state, I should decide to seek guidance, which I did and got from the kindest expert in the field. I have translated two extracts from the poem and am enclosing a copy of that translation as an expression of our thanks to you.

Praying for your happy long life and, for those you love, all the good health that a father would wish for his own ...

I didn't hear from the Luqmans again until three days before Christmas. At that time Dr. Luqman telephoned to say that Gala was attending special education classes in a local school, and that his father had returned and was now a patient at Madigan Hospital, Fort Lewis, where Dr. Luqman was stationed.

"Why, what's wrong?" I questioned, distressed by the news.

"Lung cancer, he's dying," came the laconic reply.

Shocked and greatly saddened I sent flowers — Christmas greens and white carnations. Christmas eve I had another phone call from Dr. Luqman, his father, the Poet from Yemen, was dead. Ali Luqman must have known about his illness when we met in October, I decided. Now I understood why he wrote the line 'Fear haunts me that you may suffer after my death', and why Gala was brought to America and placed in his older brother's care. I prayed that Ali's heart was at peace when he died.

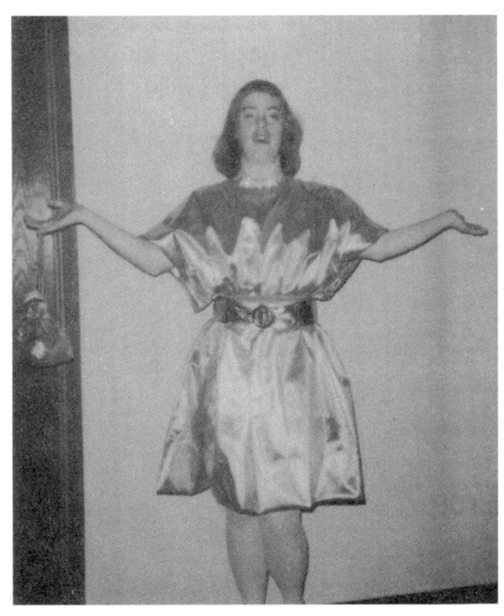

Kari singing on stage.

Chapter Thirteen
Senior Proms and Other Joys

Since 1988, like chicks hatching over a period of days from a clutch of eggs, our former Experimental Education Unit Down syndrome pupils have been cracking the shell of childhood and emerging, one by one, into the world of adults. The visible process of this emergence has been their graduation from high schools. With a few exceptions these students have been attending regular public schools, where, in addition to studying in special education classes, they were routinely included into regular classrooms with same-age pupils.

Twenty-eight years ago after I left the summer program at Fircrest I dreamed of finding a way to teach the "unreachable": of enhancing the development of disabled young children, that they might escape the fate of the abandoned ones I encountered in our state schools. When I began with the Down syndrome infants my goals were modest. I had no far reaching ambitions. I planned the program, day by day, a step at a time, never looking too far ahead. I never foresaw, in fact, that the helpless infants whom we diligently taught how to focus on objects, how to reach for playthings, how to sit, walk, speak, and eventually, read, write and count, would one day surge ahead, beyond the protective environment of the Experimental Education Unit. Their ability to do so and to emerge as victors — graduating from integrated schools — surpassed my wildest expectations.

Beyond the fact that I was willing to take a chance on these children, and beyond devising a system of early instruction that worked, I can take little credit for what happened. Although my staff and I may have sparked that first flicker of cognition that enabled our pupils to learn, the parents were the ones who fanned the flame, and who, through their demands, encouraged dedicated teachers to keep that fire burning. As we glory in our pupils' subsequent achievement we must recognize that none of this would be possible had not the potential for success existed within these children from the very beginning.

The potential exists and obviously individuals with Down syndrome are capable of achieving far more than it was ever expected of this population in the past. This is not to say, however, that education and early intervention can make these children "normal". Many medical problems can be remedied; physical, mental, language and social development can be accelerated and enhance, but the deficits inherent to this genetic anomaly can never be completely eradicated, at least not with our present medical and biochemical technology.

In 1987 I was asked to return to Japan to give another series of workshops and to present a follow-up paper on the progress of the first eleven pupils to enter the Down syndrome program in 1971. So, prior to my departure I contacted and reassessed nine of our former students. There were only nine instead of the original eleven because one member of the group left the state and B.J., one of our brightest pupils, died of of a viral infection and heart failure when she was eight.

I chose the Peabody Picture Vocabulary Test for my reassessment because it was one of the tools we used to evaluate progress during the years when the children were in our program. This choice enabled me to compare the students' present scores with those obtained in the past. One way of measuring performance is to calculate a child's mental age in reference to the chronological age. Among the normal population, according to standardized intelligence tests, such as the Stanford Binet, it is assumed that the mental age is equal to that of the chronological age. All typical twelve-year-olds, for example, are expected to function mentally at that age level, in other words, the mental age should be approximately a hundred percent of the age in years. Among the developmentally delayed population, however, we can expect to find a discrepancy between the two figures. A severely retarded twelve-year-old, for example, may be functioning mentally at the level of a three-year-old, indicating a mental age that is twenty-five percent of the chronological age.

Strictly speaking, the Peabody Picture Vocabulary Test isn't a measure of intelligence, nevertheless the scores can be analyzed to give a mental age reading. The result of my assessment was gratifying in spite of the fact that the scores of two subjects were too unreliable to include in the final analysis. Illness on the part of one individual and deafness an the part of the other precluded my using their test scores (Dmitriev, 1988). Nevertheless, ten years after their last assessment, individual scores showed that the percent of the chronological age at which these former pupils were functioning now was as high and in some cases higher than in the past. Although the mental growth of individuals with Down syndrome is slower than that of the typical population, the predicted deterioration didn't occur. At their own rate our students' mental maturity kept pace with the passing years, and the gap between their mental and chronological ages didn't widen, as it would have had their mental capabilities ceased developing. This in fact has been the argument held by some educators who question the viability of early intervention, claiming that children with Down syndrome are unable to develop intellectually after age five. Those of us who believe otherwise, are pleased to learn that this need not be the case.

DENNIS*

Dennis was one of our former students whose test score couldn't be included in the results that I obtained. Regretfully, Dennis, our beloved fair-haired, happy infant whose hearing deteriorated so rapidly in preschool, was unable, due to his severe hearing loss, to complete the Peabody Test and as a result I couldn't make an accurate analysis of his ability. It was a big disappointment and it saddened me to realize to what degree deafness limited his performance. I should have been prepared, however. A few years back when it came time for Dennis and his Down syndrome classmates to enter an integrated middle school which served normal as well as a few developmentally delayed pupils, capable of functioning in that environment, Dennis was left behind. Hampered by his hearing loss and no longer able to keep up, Dennis was enrolled in a segregated special education school. Under the circumstances this was a realistic placement. The classes were small and more emphasis was placed upon vocational training than academic instruction.

When I saw Dennis in 1987 he was nineteen years old. In spite of his extremely limited speech and shyness, I found him to be a gentle, responsive, attractive young man with the same, sweet, sunny smile he had as a child. Although somewhat short in stature, Dennis is well proportioned and exceptionally well-coordinated. He participates in Special Olympics and has won many prizes for his running ability.

The year after our meeting, Dennis went to live at the New Hope Farm, a communal living program for handicapped people, sponsored by a religious organization. The Farm is located in Goldendale, a small agricultural community in Eastern Washington. His mother reports that Dennis is very happy and thoroughly enjoys all aspects of the program; work, recreation, church services and religious instruction. The first year that Dennis was there, he attended the Goldendale High School. He graduated with normal peers in a small heartwarming ceremony the following June.

During the day the New Hope Farm residents work at various jobs in the community. They are housed in five separate three-bedroom mobile homes, four residents to a cottage, two to a room. The third bedroom is occupied by the supervising house-parents. Dennis shares a room with a developmentally disabled non-Down syndrome young man with whom he has a close and satisfying friendship.

KARI

Consistently, over the years, Kari's high scores on the Peabody and similar tests approached normalcy. Today, even though Kari lost all function of her thyroid gland and must rely on daily medication in order to maintain adequate thyroid levels, she continues to function extremely well.

While in high school Kari lettered in swimming as a member of the swimming team. Now, with school days behind her, Kari lives independently in a house which she shares with four other women, three of whom are developmentally delayed. Kari is relatively tall, slender with an attractive figure and auburn hair. She has excellent speech and participates in many social and physical activities. She enjoys folk dancing, plays the piano and sings. She also swims and skis. The summer before graduation Kari and three other girls, former EEU pupils who were not included in the follow-up study, spent four weeks working at a summer camp. They cleaned, painted and did general maintenance work. Currently Kari is employed by the Puget Consumers CO-OP where she has worked for a number of years.

PATRICK*

Patrick was the first fledgling to graduate. He completed his education at the Eastside Catholic High School in Bellevue. A good-looking, gregarious young man with fair complexion and wavy black hair, he enjoyed school, made many friends and participated in a wide range of activities. As manager of the varsity football team he attended all games and travelled with the team when it played out of town. He was also on the swim team. In class Patrick studied World Culture, Religion, Language, Math, Literature, Occupational Placement and Study Skills, Typing and Computer Science.

One of Patrick's special friends is a young woman with Down syndrome who graduated from Eastside Catholic a year ahead of him. Angie was Patrick's date for the Senior Prom. They made an attractive couple; he in his tux and she in a pale blue, off-the-shoulder formal.

Patrick has many hobbies, among them making video tapes with his video camera, listening to music - everything from Mozart to Rock — and working on his word processor are his favorites. Patrick is currently employed by Microsoft. He works for the Microsoft

Audio Visual Services where he performs a variety of demanding skill-related duties.

LUPITA*, MARTHA* AND GLEN*

In May of 1990, on the night of the Nathan High Senior Prom, Mrs. Cano*, Lupita's mother planned a dinner party for her daughter and seven graduating classmates, all of whom were going to the Prom. Pat Oelwein and I were also invited and it was a big thrill for us to be present at such a happy occasion. Lupita, Martha and Glen were among the nine students that I evaluated in 1987. The trio have been close friends since early preschool. Glen and Martha have been dating since high school and plan to get married some day. Both sets of parents approve.

The other young adults at the party, including Lupita's date, were also developmentally disabled, but none had Down syndrome. Martha and Lupita wore party dresses that had long, fitted bodices and short flouncy skirts. Both carried corsages of rosebuds and baby's breath on their wrists. With their Hispanic black hair, soft and glossy, dark eyes flashing with excitement, they looked pretty and vivacious as they flirted, sweetly coquettish, with their dates. Glen, a blond boy with blue eyes, looked particularly handsome in his light gray tuxedo. His lavender cumberbund matched the ribbon in Martha's corsage. Lupita's friend, tall and dark haired, looked elegant in his traditional black-tie attire.

I wished the whole world could see how attractive and capable these young people appeared as they sat at the candle-lit table, toasting each other with sparkling cider, talking and laughing with complete social poise and good manners. For Pat and me, and for the parents who were present this was a moment of poignant happiness and pride. Future plans for Lupita and her friends center on continued vocational and academic training at a community college, competitive employment and independent living.

EPILOGUE

The most significant thing is not how much our former students have achieved, but the fact that their success stories are not unique. Everywhere I turn, I see individuals with Down syndrome and other disabilities functioning as well, if not better than many of our so-called normal persons. One example is Chris Burke, the young man with Down syndrome who starred as "Corky Thatcher" in the national TV series *Life Goes On*. Jason Kingsley*, another actor with Down syndrome, guest starred in *The Fall Guy*. Although not all people with Down syndrome become actors, Jean Edwards* (1988) a well-known professor in special education at Portland State University, has identified seventy-two jobs, ranging from aircraft shipper to wire cutter which have been successfully performed, in competitive settings, by employees with Down syndrome.

The change in attitude towards the disabled that has taken place among doctors, educators, administrators as well as the general public over the past twenty-odd years has had a tremendous effect upon the lives individuals with disabilities and is directly responsible for this burgeoning of heretofore undetected talent and ability. This is not to deny that a great deal remains to be done in terms of acceptance, education, employment and recreational opportunities, as well as accessibility to public buildings and transportation through ramps and hydraulic lifts for wheel chairs. Then too, barriers and discrimination that occur on the basis of test scores need to be eliminated.

In the final analysis test scores are not important. We have nothing, as yet, that can measure the quality of life or what a disabled person can achieve from the stand point of human dignity, social and economic worth. As I look to the future I trust the day will come when society will no longer judge a person strictly on the basis of an I.Q. or mental age score, but rather by what he is able to contribute to the human experience be it through physical labor or through the simple sharing of a gentle, loving spirit with others.

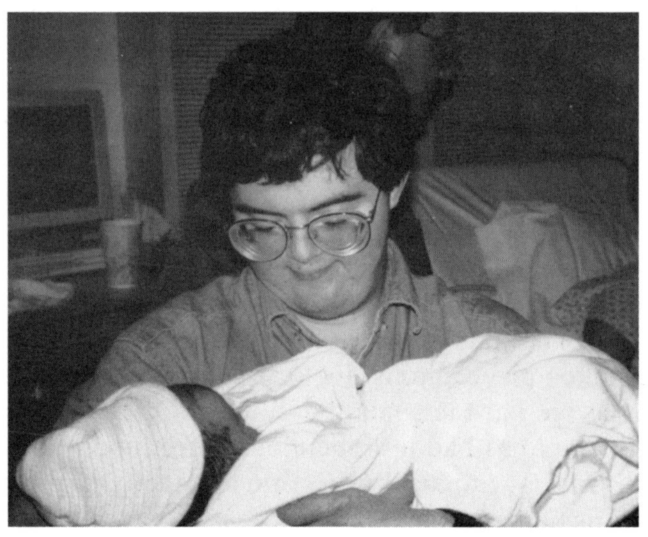

"Uncle Patrick"
Patrick holding his sister's baby.

Appendix

Resource Information through the courtesy of:
DOWN SYNDROME PROGRAM
Center on Human Development and Disability
Box 357920
University of Washington, Seattle, WA 98195-7920
Patricia Oelwein, Coordinator
Phone: 206/685-3205
FAX: 206/543-5771;
E-MAIL: oelwein@u.washington.edu

LOCAL RESOURCE LIST FOR DOWN SYNDROME

FAMILY SUPPORT AND SERVICES

The Arc of King County
10550 Lake City Way NE, Suite A.
Seattle, WA 98125
Email: the.arc@smtp.prostar.com

Administration; 206/364-6337
-Adult Services; 206/364-1613
-Advocate Resource Specialist
Kathi Whittaker; 206/364-4645
-Family Service/Parent to Parent; 206/364-6337
-Schools Are for Everyone (SAFE)
Vickie Louden (inclusion in school); 206/364-1613

Bridge Ministries for Disability Concerns
Redmond, WA; 206/882-0223
(social service and aid)

Center for Community Support
TASH (after October 1, 1995)
1932 - 1 st Avenue #905
Seattle, WA 98101

Down Syndrome Community
Seattle, WA (parent support)
Nick & Linda Kappes (N. Seattle) 206/527-2496
Linda Michael (S. Seattle) 206/241-0353
Amy & Dick Jahn (Renton) - 206/228-2385
Jane & Jeff Hall (Bellevue)206/881-6143

Birth to Three Support
Ramona Gillett (Snohomish) 206/487-9648
JoAnne Thelin (Seattle) 206/431-9777

Easter Seal Society of Washington
Seattle, WA; 206/281-5700
(information and social services)

Father's Network
Bellevue, WA; 206/747-4004

Sibling Support Project
Seattle, WA; 206/368-4911
FAX: 206/368-4816
(support and workshops for siblings of persons with disabilities)

Statewide Parent to Parent Information
800/821-5927

Washington PAVE
(Parents Are Vital in Education)
206/572-7368
Parent-To-Parent Training Project
6316 S. 12th Street, Tacoma, WA 98465-1900
206/565-2266; 800-5-PARENT; FAX: 206/566-8052
Email: wapave@nwrain.com

Washington Technology Access Center
8511 - 15th Avenue NE
Seattle, WA 98115-3199
206/526-1240 (Voice/Fax)
Internet: WTA@AppleLink.apple.com

INTERDISCIPLINARY
DIAGNOSTIC/ASSESSMENT

Center on Human Development and Disability (CHDD)
U of W, Box 357920
Seattle WA 98195-7920
206/685-1251
WWW site: http://weber.u.washington.ed~chddwww/

Children's Hospital and Medical Center (CHMC)
4800 Sand Point Way NE, Seattle WA 98105
206/526-2000

Pediatric Referral Program of King County
Seattle:206/284-0331; Toll Free: 800-756-KIDS

EARLY INTERVENTION PROGRAMS

Birth to Three Developmental Center
Federal Way, WA; 206/874-5445

Boyer Children's Clinic
Seattle, WA; 206/325-8477
(Birth to 3 Early Intervention Program)

Children's Therapy Center of Kent
Kent, WA; 206/854-5660
(Birth to 3 Early Intervention Program)

Infant and Toddler Program
Experimental Education Unit (EEU) CHDD,
University of Washington 206/543-4011

Kindering Center
Bellevue, WA; 206/747-4004
(Birth to 3 early intervention program)

Northwest Center
Seattle, WA; 206/286-2322
Birth to 5 Early Intenvention Program

RECREATIONAL PROGRAMS

Camp Easter Seal
Vaughn, WA, 206/884-2722
(good summer camps)

Emerald City Gymnastics
Bellevue, WA; 206/861-8772 (gymnastic lessons)

Highland Center
Bellevue Parks and Recreation Department
Bellevue, WA; 206/455-7686
(programs for children and adults with disabilities)

Kent Park & Recreations Department
Kent, WA, 206/859-3350
(recreational and social activities that include persons with developmental disabilities)

Little Bit Therapeutic Riding Center
Woodinville, WA; 206/882-1554
(non-profit organization serving children and adults with disabilities by providing a unique, recreational approach to therapy through the use of the horse)

Seattle Department of Parks and Recreation
Special Programs; 206/684-4950

Summer Camp Program
Stanley Stamm Children's Hospital Camp
Seattle, WA; 206/526-2267
(for children with disabilities and chronic illness)

Ski for All
Seattle, WA; 206/328-4911
(ski in winter, hike in summer)

Special Olympics
Seattle, WA; 206/362-4949

OTHER PROGRAMS AND SERVICES

Aging with Down syndrome Clinic
University of Washington
Doug Cook, 206/685-1280

Camp Fire's Special Sitters
Seattle, WA; 206/461-8550

Developmental Disabilities Community Support Project
Seattle, WA; 206/623-2814
(behavior management services and crisis intervention)

DOWN SYNDROME PROGRAM
Center on Human Development and Disability
Box 357920
University of Washington, Seattle, WA 98195-7920
Patricia Oelwein Coordinator
Phone: 206/685-3205
FAX: 206/543-5771; E-MAIL:
oelwein@u.washington.edu

King County Division of Developmental Disabilities
Seattle, WA; 206/296-5214

King County Interagency Coordinating Council
Glen Fetion; 206/720-3331

King County Parent Coalition
for Developmental Disabilities
Margaret Lee Thompson;
206/296-5214
(special programs)

People First
Chapters Statewide, 800-758-1123
(adult self-advocacy group)

Washington Division of Developmental Disabilities
Seattle, 206/464-5488 & 720-3300
Spokane, 509/456-2893

Sundial Travel
600 Broadway
Seaside, OR 97138
800-547-9198
(Chaperoned tours for people with developmental disabilities)

Washington Academy of Performing Arts:
Extraordinary Program
Redmond, WA; 206/556-9693
(performing arts for children with special needs, inclusive and special programs)

Siblings Information Network Newsletter CUAP
991 Main Street, East Hartford, CT 06108
$15/year; 4 issues (for siblings of children with disabilities, not specific to Down syndrome)

NATIONAL RESOURCES LIST FOR DOWN SYNDROME

National Organizations
The ARC (National)
2501 Avenue J, Arlington, TX 76006;
817/640-0204

National Down syndrome Congress
1605 Chantilly Drive, Suite 250, Atlanta, GA 30324
800/232-NDSC; 404/633-1555 (GA)
E-mail: ndsc@charitiesusa.com
WWW address: http://www.carol.net/~ndsc/

National Down syndrome Society 666 Broadway,
New York, NY 10012
800/221-4602; 212/460-9330

Siblings for Significant Change
105 East 22nd Street, New York, NY 10010
212/420-0776

Siblings Information Network, CUAP
991 Main Street, East Hartford, CT 06108
203/282-7050

TASH (The Association for the Severely Handicapped)
29 W. Susquehanna Avenue, Suite 210
Baltimore, MD 21204
410/828-8274; Fax: 410-828-6706
TDD: 410-828-1360; 800-463-5685
Fax: 905-686-6895

Books Available from:
Brookes Publishing Company
P.O. Box 10624
Baltimore, MD 21285-9945
800/638-3775

Biomedical Concerns in Persons with Down syndrome Edited by S.M. Pueschel and J.K. Pueschel (1992) ($43.00)

Brothers, Sisters, and Special Needs By D. J. Lobato (I 990) ($28. 00)

Choosing Options and Accommodations for Children (COACIO: A Guide for Planning Inclusive Education) By M.F. Giangreco, C. J. Cloninger & V. S. Iverson (1992) ($29.00)

New Perspective on Down syndrome
Edited by S.M. Pueschel, C. Tingey, J.E. Rynders, A.C. Crocker, D.M. Crutcher (1986) ($32.95)

A Parent's Guide to Down syndrome
By S. M. Pueschel (1990) ($20.00)

Sibshops, Workshops for Siblings of Children with Special Needs
By D. J. Meyer and P. F. Vadasy (1994) $32.00

The Syracuse Community-Referenced Curriculum Guide for Students with Moderate and Severe Disabilities
Edited by A. Ford, R. Schnorr, L. Meyer, L. Davem, J.Black and P. Dempsey (1989, $47.00)

Books Available from:
PRO-ED
8700 Shoal Creek Boulevard
Austin, TX 78758-9965
312/451-3246; FAX 512/451-8542

My Friend, David
By J. Edwards and D. Dawson (1983) ($12.00)

Teaching the Infant with Down syndrome. A Guide for Parents and Professionals
By M. Hanson (1986) ($22.00)

Teaching the Young Child with Motor Delays: A Guide for Parents and Professionals
By. A Hanson and S. Harris (1986) ($21.00)

Books Available from:
University of Washington Press
P.O. Box, C-50096
Seattle, WA 98145-5096
800-638-3775

A Handbook for the Fathers Program
By D.J. Meyer, P.F. Vadasy, & R.R. Fewell (1985) ($24.95)

Grandparent Workshops: How to Organize Workshops for Grandparents of Children with Handicaps
By D.J. Meyer, P.F. Vadasv, & R.R. Fewell (1986) ($14.95)

Living with a Brother or Sister with Special Needs: A Book for Sibs
By D.J. Meyer & P.F.Vadasy (1996)

Books Available from:
Woodbine House
6510 Bells Mill Road
Bethesda, NM 20817
800/843-7323; FAX 301/897-5838

Babies with Down syndrome; Second Edition
By Karen Stray-Gundersen (1995) ($15.95)

Communication Skills in Children with Down syndrome: A Guide for Parents
By L. Kumin (1994) ($14.95)

Differences in Common
By M. Trainer (1991) ($14.95)
(collection of essays about raising a child with Down syndrome)

The Language of Toys: Teaching Communication Skills to Special-Needs Children a Guide for Parents and Teachers
By S. Schwartz & J.E.H. Miller (1988) ($14.95)

Medical & Surgical Care for Children with Down syndrome: A Guide for Parents
Edited by D.C. Van Dyke, P. Mattheis, S. Eberly, and J. Williams (1995) ($14.95)

Teaching Reading to Children with Down syndrome: A Guide for Parents and Teachers
By P. L. Oelwein (1995) ($16.95)

Uncommon Fathers: Reflections on Raising a Child with a Disability
Edited by D.J. Meyer (1995) ($14.95)

Periodicals
The Arc
National Headquarters
2501 Avenue J, Austin TX 76006; 817/604-0204
$15/year - 6 issues
The Arc comes with the $15 membership in the National Arc)

Communicating Together
The Institute for Effective Communication Skills
P.O. Box 6395
Columbia, MD 21045-6395

Annual subscription rate for 6 issues is $20 in US, $25 in US funds; outside USA.
Make check or money order payable to:
Communicating Together.
(A newsletter for parents and professional about speech and language skills in children with Down syndrome.)

Communicating Partners
P.O. Box 141306
Columbus, OH 43202
$15 per year 4 issues
(A newsletter for parents of children developing language, edited by Barbara Mitchell and James D. MacDonald)

Disability Solutions
9220 S.W. Barbur Blvd. # 119-179
Portland, OR 97219
503/244-7662
(Published 6 times a year by The Enoch-Gelbard Foundation; free and informative.)

Down syndrome News
Membership Services, NDSC
1605 Chantilly Drive, Suite 250, Atlanta, GA 30324
$20/year, 10 issues; outside U.S.A. add $10
(comes with
NDSC membership).

Down syndrome Quarterly
Samuel J. Thios, Ph.D., Editor
Granville, Ohio 43023
Individual subscriptions: $24, one year; $48 two years Library/Organization: $48, one year; $90, two years (Orders outside US: Canada & Mexico, add $6 per year, other foreign order add $10 per year, payment must be made in US funds and must accompany orders.)

Down syndrome Quarterly (cont)
(Journal devoted to advancing the state of knowledge on Down syndrome — covers all areas of medical, behavioral, and social scientific research.)

News 'n Views, N.D.S. S.
666 Broadway
New York, NY 10012-2317
800/221-4602
$10/year, 3 issues per year
(A magazine written by and for teenagers and adults with Down syndrome)

The Exceptional Parent
P.O. Box 3000,
Dept. EP,
Denville, NJ 07834-9919
$28year, 12 issues (for parents of children with disabilities, not specific to Down syndrome)

National Association of Sibling Programs Newsletter
Sibling Support Project, CL-09, CHMC
4800 Sand Point Way NE,
Seattle WA 98105

Books Available from:
John Wiley, Inc.
605 Third Ave, New York, NY 10 158-0012
800-225-5945

Down syndrome: Advances in Medical Care
Edited by Irs T. Lott & Ernest E. McCoy
(1992) ($24.95)

Down syndrome: Living and Learning in the Community
Edited by L. Nadel & D. Rosenthal (1995)($17.95)

Books Available from Other Publishers:

Becoming Partners with Children: From Play to Conversation
By J.D. MacDonald
Riverside Publishing Company ($31.50)
8420 Bryn Marr Avenue, Suite 1000
Chicago, U, 60631 (800/232-9540)

Children with Down syndrome: A Development Perspective
Edited by D. Cicchetti & M. Beeghly
Cambridge University Press (1990) ($19.95)
40 West 20th Street, New York, NY 10011

Circles of Friends
By R. Perske
Abingdon Press (1988)
201 Eighth Avenue S.
Nashville, TN 37202

Count Us In; Growing up with Down syndrome
By J. Kingsley and M. Levitz
Harcourt Brace & Company (1994) ($9.95)
15 East 26th Street, New York, NY 10010

Down syndrome (Pamphlet)
NDSC Central Office
1605 Chantilly Drive, Atlanta GA 30324
100 for $70.00; $0.75 each

Down syndrome: Birth to Adulthood: Giving Families an EDGE
By John E. Rynders & Jim Horrobin (1995)
Love Publishing Company ($29.95)
1777 S. Bellaire St
Denver, CO 80222
(303/757-2579)

Down syndrome: The Facts
By Mark Selikowitz
Oxford University Press (1990) ($20.95)
200 Madison Ave, New York, NY 10016
800/451-7556

Down's Syndrome: Psychological, Psychobiological and Socio-Educational Perspectives
Edited by J.A.Rondal, J. Perera, L.Nadel, and A.Comblain Whurr Publishers Ltd (1996)
19b Compton Terrace, London NI 2UN, England

It Takes Two to Talk: A Hanen Early Language Parent Guide
By A. Manolson
Hanen Early Language Resource Center (1983) ($34.30 in Canadian currency; money order, or VISA) 252 Bloor Street West, Toronto, Ontario M5S-IV5, Canada; 416/921-1073

Medical Care in Down syndrome: A Preventive Medical Approach
By NC Coleman and P. Rogers
Marcel Dekker, Inc.
270 Madison Avenue, New York, NY 100 16

Precious Lives, Painful choices
By Sherokee Ilse
Wintergreen Press (1993) ($7.50)
P.O. Box 165, Long Lake MN 55356

A Special Kind of Hero
By C. Burke and J. B. McDaniel Doubleday (1991) ($18.00)

Time to Begin
By V. Dmitriev
Penn Cove Press (1992) ($17.00)
3748 S. Oceanside Dr., Greenbank, WA 98253-9745
206/678-3209

This Baby Needs You Even More (pamphlet) National Down syndrome Society ($1. 50 each)
666 Broadway, New York, NY 10012
800/221-4602; NY only, 212/764-3070

Understanding Down syndrome
By C. Cunningham
Brookline Books (1995) ($14.95)
P.O. Box 1047, Cambridge, MA 02239
800/666-BOOK
800/229-1160

When Slow is Fast Enough
By J. Goodman
Guilford Publications ($17.95)
72 Spring Street
New York, NY 10012 (212/431-9800)

Working Together: Workplace Culture, Supported Employment and Persons with Disabilities
By D. Hagner & D. Dileo
Brookline Books (1993) ($24.95)

<u>VHS Color Videotapes Available from:</u>
Media Services
CHDD Box 357925
University of Washington
Seattle, WA 98195-7925
206/5434011

Learning on the Go ($135; 23 minutes)
This videocassette describes the way in which professionals and parents of children with disabilities can take advantage of the variety of learning opportunities that occur throughout the child's day.

Like an Ordinary Brother: The Cares of Siblings ($135; 20 minutes) Five brothers and sisters of individuals with handicaps talk with each other about their cares and concerns about a "special" sibling. Despite age, birth order, and sex differences, the group members share many common experiences and feelings.

My Turn, Your Turn ($135; 24 minutes)
Describes strategies parents and caregivers can use to foster enjoyable and successful interactions with prelinguistic infants with handicaps. This video demonstrates actual patterns that may be used to develop social and language skills in very young children.

Thanks Mom and Dad: Profiles of Patrick
($143; 33 minutes)
Through the use of videotapes, photographs, and interviews, this presentation profiles Patrick, a young man with Down syndrome, from preschool to post graduation. Patrick represents a new generation of persons with Down syndrome who have received the benefits of a nurturing home, early intervention, and challenging educational opportunities.

<u>Video Available from</u>
<u>American Film and Video Company:</u>
6900 Wisconsin Ave. Suite 206
Bethesda, MD 20815
(301) 652-1477
Roots and Wings (1995; 36 min.)

<u>Video Available from Utah Down syndrome Foundation:</u>
Southern Utah Chapter
1035 E. 100 So., SL
George, UT 84770 (800-773-0437)

Up with Downs: A Love Story
($10.00 plus $5.00 postage, 30 minutes)
Two life stories, eventually joined as one in marriage, are told in this inspiring video.

<u>Video Available from Exceptional Parent Magazine Library:</u>
800/535-1910
Potty Learning for Children Who Experience Delay
($39)

INTERNET RESOURCES

ADOPTION ARTICLE (by Janet Marchese)
http://ptolemy.eecs.berkeley.edu/~pino/DS/news/sjmercury/adoption31596,html

THE ARC'S HOME PAGE, WWW site
http:/www.metronet.com/~thearc/welcome.html
http:/TheArc.org/welcome.html

ASSOCIATION FOR CHILDREN WITH DS
http://www.macroserve.com/acds/acdshome.htm

AXIS CONSULTATION & TRAINING
http://www.almanac.bc.ca/~axis/
Norman Kunc & Emma Van der Klift
normemma@port.island.net

BREASTFEEDING ADVOCACY
http://www.clark.net/pub/activist/bfpage/html
Australian Breastfeeding Tips
http://www.vicnet.net.au/vicnet/nmaa/downsynd.htm

CENTRAL FLORIDA DS ASSOCIATION
http://www.sundial.net/~mwinwood/cfdsa/cfdsa.htm

CHASER (Congenital Heart Anomalies: Support, Education and Resources)
http:/wwwcsu.edu/~hfmth006/sheri/heart.html
myer1O6@wonder.em.edc.gov
75050.2742@compuserve.com

THE COMMUNITY INSTITUTE
(British Columbia)
http://www.geocities.com/Athens/4820/
wetherow@qb.island.net

COUNT US IN: GROWING UP WITH DOWN SYNDROME
(Jason Kingsley & Mitchell Levitz)
http://brugold.com/count.html

DAN'S PAGE: PERSPECTIVE OF A 15 YEAR OLD WITH DOWN SYNDROME
http://members.aol.com/suebd/dance/dan.html

DOWN SYNDROME LIST SERVICE (from Pam Wilson)
To subscribe, send message to:
LISTERV@LISTERV.NODAK.EDU
with the Subject of No Subject and a message of subscribe down-syn <put your first and last name here> respond OK to the confirmation message.

You may leave the list at any time by sending a "SIGNOFF DOWN-SYN" command to
LISTERV@LISTSERV.NODAK.EDU
Once subscribed you may change your method of reading the list by sending a message <set down-syn digest>to the list service address, and all the posts will arrive in one piece of email once a day. To

unsubscribe from the digest, the message would read
<signoff down syn digest>
To send message to other parents and concerned professionals, write to

DOWN-SYN@LISTSERV.NODAK.EDU
(from PowerLine)
To send message: DOWW-SYN@vml.nodak.edu
To subscribe: SUBSCRIBE DOWN-SYN<your name>

DOWN SYNDROME WWW HOME PAGE AT URL
http://www.nas.com/downsyn/dshm.html

DOWN SYNDROME WWW HOME PAGE LINKS
http://@.nas.com/downsyn/netl.html

DOWN SYNDROME QUARTERLY page at IFRL (updated preventive medical check list) http:/www.denison.edu/dsq/health/96.html

FAMILY VILLAGE PROJECT (diverse diagnoses)
http://www.familyvillage.wisc.edu/
rowley@waisman.wisc.edu

GOLD COAST DOWN SYNDROME HOME PAGE
http://www.gate.net/~sbonsett/gcds/gcds_hme.htm

INCLUSION HOME PAGE
http://www.inclusion.com

INSTITUTE ON COMMUNITY INTEGRATION
http:/@.coled.umn.edu/iciwww/
(linked from the DS WWW page)

JAPAN DS NETWORK
http://ss.niah.affrc.go.jp/~momotani/dowj1-e.htmi

LIFE GOES ON'S ANDREA FRIEDMAN
http://www.abilitymagazin.com/ability/text/andreais.htm

NATIONAL DOWN SYNDROME CONGRESS
NDSC@charitiesusa.com
http://www.carol.net/~ndsc

NATIONAL DOWN SYNDROME SOCIETY
http://www.pcsltd.com/ndss/

OPEN WINDOW (welcoming babies with DS)
ftp://wonder.mit.edu/pub/ok/WBwDS.txt
ftp://wonder.mit.edu/pub/ok/TFtMotN.txt

Online support: pmwilson,@aol.com

OUR-KIDS WWW ARCHIVE
(former postings of the OurKids list service; diverse diagnoses) http://wonder.mit.edu/our-kids.html

PACIFIC NORTHWEST UPSIDE! SOCIETY
http://www.telebyte.com/upside/upside.html

PAVE
http://www.nwrain.net/~wapave/
wapave@nwrain.com
stomp@nwrain.com
barbara540@aol.com

SAN FRANCISCO BAY AREA DS PAGE
http://ptolemy.eecs.berkeley.edu/~pino/DS/index.html
(Includes links to a number of DS informational sites.)

SIBLING SUPPORT PROJECT
http:/www.chmc.org/departmt/sibsupp

THE SibNet LISTSERVE
Email-type bulletin board for brothers and sisters; for free subscription visit Sibling Support Project web page (see above)

TASH
email: tash@tash.org
Nancy Weiss, Executive Director
nweiss@tash.org

TIDEWATER DS ASSOCIATION (VA)
http:/www.infi.net~jwheaton/tdsahome.html
http:/www.infi.net/~jwheaton/dsnet.html (pw)

WA ASSISTIVE TECHNOLOGY ALLIANCE
http:/weber.u.washington.edu/~atrc/
uwat@u.washington.edu

WHEN (Washington Home Education Network)
(for WA Homeschoolers email list)
FmlyLrngEx@aol.com

End Notes

1. Child Development and Mental Retardation Center (CDMRC): renamed Center on Human Development and Disability (CHDD)

2. Cordocentisis: A new, less invasive prenatal screening procedure, based upon umbilical blood sampling is currently replacing amniocentisis and chorionic villi sampling. Under ultrasonographic visualization blood is drawn from the umbilical vein at its entrance to the placenta or the fetal abdominal wall.

3. Mary Janes: As a rule this type of footwear was discouraged because the soles of these shoes are apt to be stiff and slippery making it uncomfortable and dangerous for little girls when they engaged in gross motor activities such as running, climbing and even walking. Maggie, like her classmates, usually wore sneakers. On this particular day, however, when Maggie was going to meet her future adoptive mother, Betty Daniels had apparently decided to disregard this rule.

4. Language Development: Children with Down syndrome do indeed have language delays, yet as with all children the rate of language acquisition is variable and depends on many factors. Innate ability, cognitive development, general health and the frequency or infrequency of colds and middle ear infections influence the onset of speech. Adult interaction that focuses on sound and word production and overall communication skills also plays a major role in language development. Parents and teachers are now taking a much more active role in promoting speech. Consequently many more children with Down syndrome begin speaking at an earlier age than they did when we first began exploring the potential of this population twenty-five years ago.

5. Mrs. Buhler: We learned later that in addition to depriving Maggie of fluids, Mrs. Buhler put the child on a "diet", considering Maggie "too fat."

6. Bribery: A distinction must be made between bribery which is an illegal and immoral act and a reward which symbolizes recognition for a job well done.

7. Research: Operant procedures in remedial speech and language. H.N. Sloan and B.D. MacAulay (Eds.) Boston: Houghton Mifflin Co., 1968

8. Jerry: Learning to sit still long enough to fill a peg board was a major achievement for Jerry and the first step in what would have been a series of developmental tasks leading him to more age-appropriate activities with the focus on teaching him academic, functional, vocational and recreational skills. Since the Pilot program ended before Jerry returned to school, the responsibility of teaching these tasks was left in the hands of other teachers.

9. Fathers: This program has become nationwide. For more information please refer to Resources listed in the Appendix.

Dr. Valentine Dmitriev is available to conduct presentations, seminars or workshops.
For a list of suggested topics and other information, please contact:

Peanut Butter Publishing
(206) 281-5965
226 2nd Ave. W.
Seattle, WA 98119

References

Dmitriev, V. (1982) *Time to Begin,* Milton, WA; Caring, Inc. Reprinted (1992) Greenbank, WA: Penn Cove Press.

Dmitriev, V. (1988) Cognition and the acceleration and maintenance of developmental gains among children with Down syndrome: longitudinal data. Down syndrome: Papers and Abstractsfor the Professionals, January. 11, 1.

Dunn, L.M. (1959) Peabody Picture Vocabulary Test, Circle Pines, MN: American Guidance Service.

Edwards, J. (1988) Strategies for meeting the needs of adolescents and adults. In V. Dmitriev and P. Oelwein, (Eds.) Advances in Down syndrome, Seattle, WA: Special Child Publications.

Meyer, D. J. (1995) Uncommon fathers, Bethesda, MD; Woodbine House.

Oelwein, P. (1995) Teaching reading to children with Down syndrome, Bethesda, MD: Woodbine House.

Order Form

To order additional copies of:

Tears and Triumphs

please send $22.00 plus $2.50
Shipping & Handling,
Washington residents please include 8.2% sales tax.
Make check or money order payable to:

Peanut Butter Publishing
226 2nd Ave W.
Seattle, WA 98119
(206) 281-5965

If you prefer to use VISA or Mastercard, please fill in your card's number and expiration date. Please circle appropriate card.

□ □□□□□□□□□□□□□□□□

Signature________________________________

exp. date_______

______Copies @ $22.00 ea.________
$2.50 Shipping & Handling________
Washington State residents add 8.2%_______
Total enclosed_______

Name________________________________
Address________________________________
City, State, Zip________________________________

Standard Discounts available.
Please list additional copies to be sent to other addresses on a separate sheet.

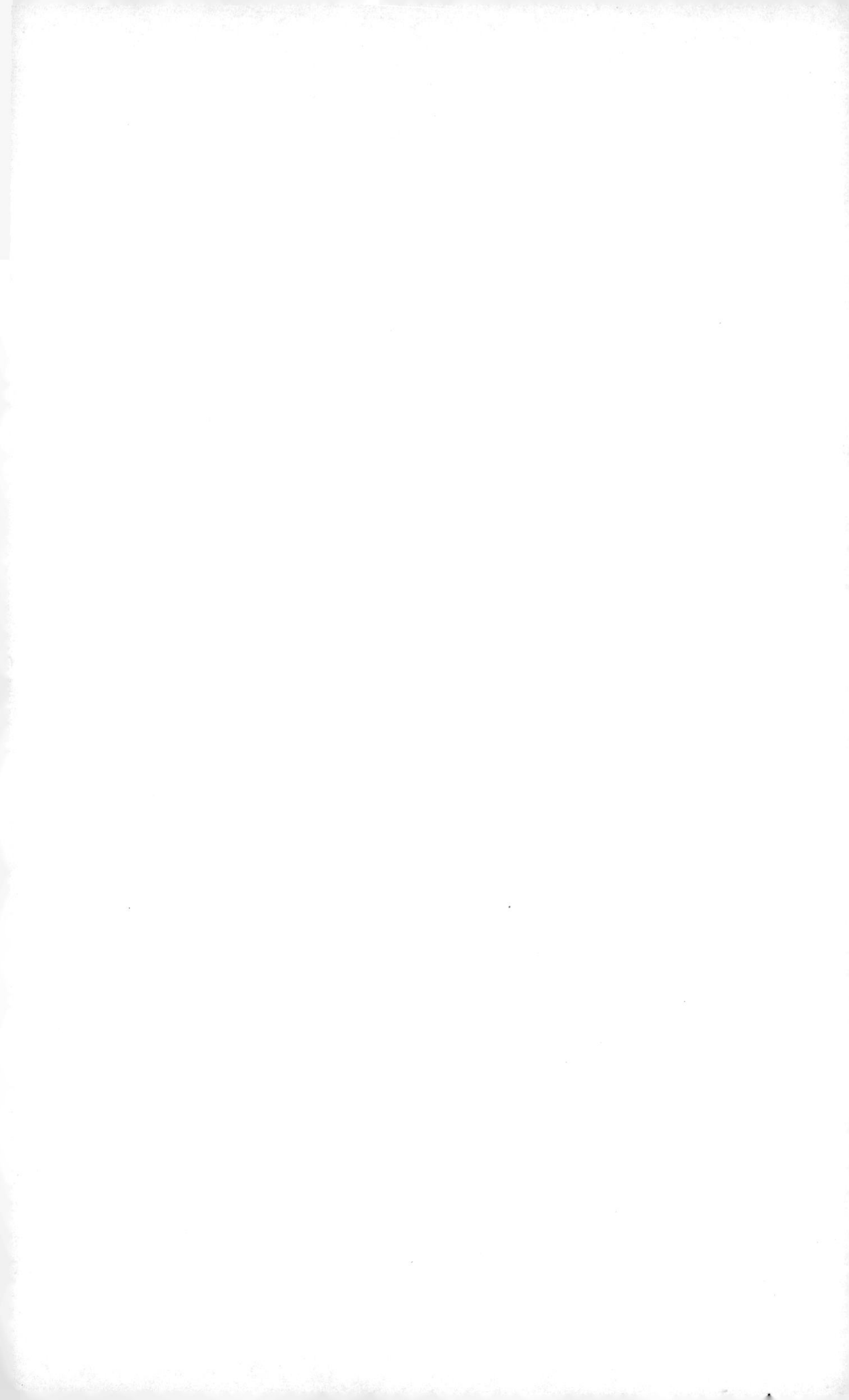